COVID-19!

COVID-19!

How You Can
Lower Your Risk
During the Pandemic

A Virologist

Answers Questions

Shares Facts

Offers Advice

By Clyde R. Goodheart, MD, MBA, MS
And
Barbara Goodheart, BA, ELS

ISBN 978-1-994084-02-8

Notice to readers

COVID-19! How You Can Lower Your Risk During the Pandemic is distributed with the understanding that the authors and publisher are not rendering medical advice for COVID-19 or any other health condition. This ebook is intended only for general information about SARS-CoV-2 and the disease it causes, COVID-19, its risks to you, and suggestions on how to evaluate those risks. Patients should consult their health care professionals for medical advice.

Contents

Introduction

This book is about you. The risks you face during this awful pandemic. What you can do to protect your health and the health of those you care about.

This book is not about, or for, those who ignore the guidelines for protecting themselves and others from COVID-19. Or what countries should do to combat the pandemic. Or what politicians should or should not do to reopen their economies. Or about mistakes our political leaders made and are making, or how we could have prevented many of the problems COVID-19 caused.

People want to resume living as we did before the pandemic. And governments—local, state, federal—want that too, to reboot the world's economy. Yet the time to return to life as it was hasn't yet come, although it may arrive soon. So when government officials decide it's all right for us to stop following the guidelines—wearing masks, social distancing, and handwashing—or to go back to restaurants and bars or to church or to work, ask yourself, "Am I ready for that? Does that advice feel right for me? Do I want to take that risk?"

Because you do have choices.

Some risks are unavoidable. Others you can choose to sidestep.

In the mood for a carryout meal from your favorite restaurant? Researchers rank that as low risk, at the far bottom of the risk scale.

Tempted to go to the barbershop or hair stylist? You might want to rethink that one. (There's a reason many COVID-19 experts on television are seriously in need of a haircut and color treatment.) The risk level varies, depending on the protective measures the shop is taking, but the risk tends to be right up there with having drinks at a bar.

Some risks you may need to take. If a close relative thousands of miles away is seriously ill, you may need to fly there. Researchers rank flying as medium risk, but it can be highly risky if you don't take the right precautions. We let you know what those precautions are, so you can fly as safely as possible.

In short, you do have choices in this pandemic. You can get the information to keep your risk at a minimum.

Ready to start?

Decide what's important to you, and carry it through

- See if your choices carry a low, medium, or high risk
- Find out what you can do to lower those risks
- Make your choices
- Put our advice and suggestions to work

We'll help you evaluate the risks and keep them as low as possible.

Protect yourself

Now that we have vaccines, take advantage of the protection they provide. Get vaccinated as soon as your turn comes up.

Clyde R. Goodheart, MD, MBA, MS
Fort Lauderdale, Florida 33308
June 2021

What's in This Book

The book has a simple format: a collection of questions family members and friends have asked me about COVID-19 and the virus that causes it, and my answers.

I worked with my wife, Barbara, also a medical writer and Certified Editor in the Life Sciences (ELS), in drafting answers for many of those questions. Barbara also developed our extensive Glossary.

Whenever possible I've structured the answers so that a simple explanation comes right up, and, for those who want it—and many do, I've found—detailed information and perhaps suggestions and reassurances follow.

We've inserted a row of asterisks at the beginning and end of detailed sections. So when you see ************* you can skip that section if you're not interested in additional detail. An index to all the questions is at the back of the book so you can quickly find the ones you're interested in.

Whenever a good reference source has turned up, I've included it. In all cases I've based the answers on the most reliable, most recent information I could find at that time.

But here's something we know all too well in medical science: often, as data accumulate, we learn, sometimes to our delight, sometimes to our embarrassment, sometimes even to our chagrin, that some things that we thought were true, probably aren't. Or they're partly true. Or they're flat-out wrong.

Being a scientist means being willing to change viewpoints when better information comes along. That's inevitable while learning about a virus and receiving new information almost daily from leading scientists and doctors around the world. Even world-renowned experts like Dr. Anthony Fauci, director of the National Institute of Allergy and Infectious Diseases, have changed their opinions on occasion based on new information.

Yet some people have slammed COVID-19 experts who have the courage to state their opinions without always tempering them with "to the best of our knowledge at the moment . . . " then later, when new data come out, need to change their statements. Unfortunately, some people have lost confidence in medical experts as a result.

Writing this book has been challenging. Sometimes as soon as an answer to a question was written, credible new information came in that changed the answer. Sometimes the question and answer became obsolete, and we deleted it.

We also expect that as soon as we publish this book, certain parts will be obsolete. So please bear with us. We'll try to keep our website up to date as information changes; if appropriate, we'll also bring this book up to date in a second edition.

The speed and extent of acquiring new information of this magnitude has never been seen before. We consider this to be a healthy situation, despite the difficulties it puts on authors like us.

Prologue

The COVID-19 year 2020 was terrible beyond belief. Cases, deaths—totals that seemed impossible in early spring of 2020 became a reality.

People have always had a deep fear of pandemics. "Will I be the next to die?" is a rational question; a quick look back in history shows why. The Black Death plague that hit Europe, Asia, and Africa in the mid-14th century raged for four years, killing an estimated 200 million people—almost half the population of medieval Europe.

With fewer people to feed, European food prices dropped. Labor markets changed. Previously impoverished survivors of the plague inherited land and gained political power—changes still evident today.

More than four centuries later, the Spanish flu pandemic of 1918 broke out, infecting about 550 million people worldwide—almost one-third of the world's population at that time. The losses were devastating. At least one of every 30 to 35 people died, with some estimates putting total deaths at 50 million to 100 million.

During a two-year rampage in the U.S., the Spanish flu killed about 675,000 people—out of a population of about 103 million—then abruptly ended. Total U.S. deaths exceeded those in World War I, World War II, the Korean War, and the Vietnam War combined.

The current global scourge, caused by a new virus, SARS-CoV-2, was declared a pandemic in early 2020. For many people, it brought months of misery and isolation. For many, death.

But things have changed since early 2020. Today, we know much more about the virus. We know effective ways to protect ourselves, and we have vaccines. And doctors have more tools for treating COVID-19 patients.

The reasons:

- *Research findings* are yielding useful data about how the COVID-19 virus acts and multiplies, and how COVID-19 develops and spreads.
- *Clinical trials* rapidly provide data on life-saving treatments. Unlike the trials of a half-century ago, with what we now consider faulty designs, modern trials yield robust, unbiased, highly useable data.
- *The internet* and related electronic capabilities rapidly process COVID-19 information and distribute it worldwide.

And yet, the disease and death totals from COVID-19 continued to rise in 2020 and into 2021.

Early on, the U.S. government saw the need for a vaccine and provided massive funding for researchers and pharmaceutical companies. No one knew which of the competitors might win the vaccine race or even if a vaccine was possible for this virus. Drug companies quickly gathered their resources and worked in parallel. Gifted researchers, given freedom, followed their instincts; in an unprecedented move, the government, not the companies, accepted the huge financial risks.

In December 2020, just as the number of COVID-19 cases and deaths were hitting the highest levels since the beginning of the pandemic, two pharmaceutical companies *announced FDA had granted emergency use authorization (EUA) for their highly effective vaccines—vaccines created at a speed never before seen in the history of vaccine development.*

We now know how to avoid COVID-19, how to treat it, and how to prevent it. COVID-19 patients are getting better medical care than ever before, and their risk of dying has dropped sharply.

And we know some reasons for the huge surge in cases that overwhelmed the health care system in December 2020.

Holiday visits and family get-togethers almost certainly played a major role, as did premature opening of restaurants and bars. But throughout the year, as quarantine fatigue grew, ignoring the three key guidelines in effect before the vaccines: wearing a mask, keeping at least a six-foot distance, and washing hands for 20 seconds, were the most important causes of COVID-19 cases and deaths.

The vaccines have proven to be highly effective and safe; being vaccinated is far safer than not being vaccinated. Now nearly all people being hospitalized with COVID-19 are people who haven't been vaccinated.

But the pandemic, unfortunately, is not over.

When unvaccinated people become infected with the coronavirus, increased viral replication allows new variants to appear. It's quite possible that some new variants will evade the current vaccines. If so, we'll need new vaccines. And we'll have another round of vaccinations. And many who do not get vaccinated will die.

It's also possible that the current pandemic could end as the 1918 flu pandemic may have. But did it? According to the influenza and infectious disease experts, Drs. Morens, Taubenberger, and Fauci, the flu pandemic never did end. Instead, each year it returns in a new guise: that of the much milder seasonal flu.

Each year's influenza viruses are genetically traceable to the 1918 virus. Unless we're lucky, this could happen with the current COVID-19 pandemic—we might have to learn to live with SARS-CoV-2 and its descendants.

And now let's move on to the Questions and Answers.

What is a Virus?

FIVE VIRUSES: BEAUTIFUL, BUT DEADLY

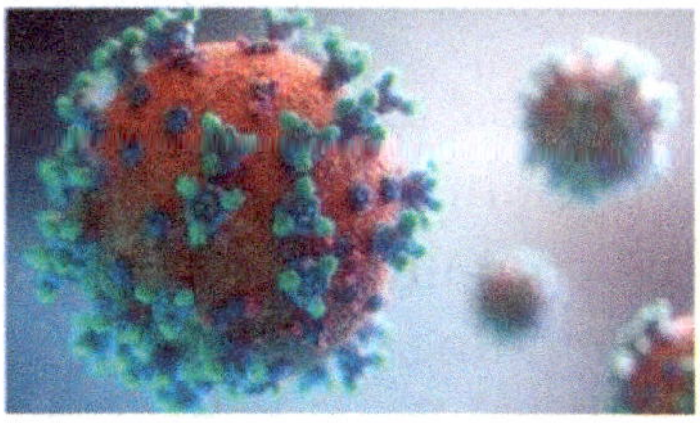

Spanish Flu H1N1 Pandemic —1918 – 1920— World: 550 million cases, 50-100 million deaths CFR: 0.1 – 5.0%; R_0 = 2.0	2009 H1N1 Influenza A (Swine Flu) Pandemic —1918 – 1920— US: 60.8 million cases, 12,469 deaths CFR: less than 1%; R_0 = 2.0

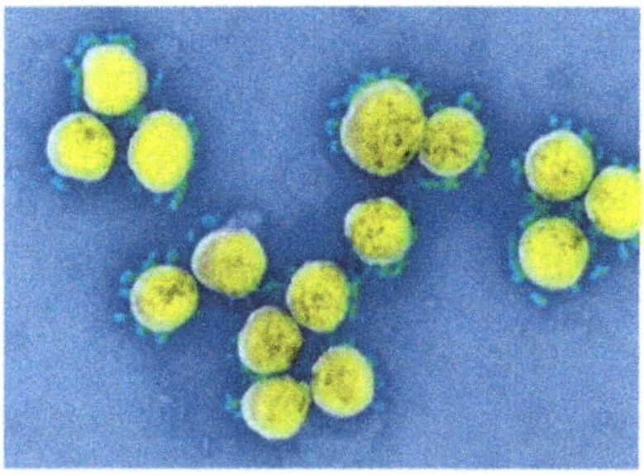

SARS-CoV – Severe acute respiratory syndrome coronavirus — 2003 — (outbreak) World: 8,096 cases, 774 deaths CFR: 9.6%; R_0 = 2.0	MERS-CoV—Middle East respiratory syndrome coronavirus — 2012 — (outbreak) World: 2,424 cases, 858 deaths CFR: 34%; R_0 = 0.9

SARS-CoV-2 — Severe acute
respiratory syndrome coronavirus
— 2019 - ? — (pandemic)
As of 3-18-2021, in US:
29.6 million cases, 538 thousand deaths
CFR: 1.8%; R_0 = less than 1 for 42 states

COVID-19!

At the bottom of this deadly pandemic: a tiny entity called a virus

An individual virus unit is commonly called a virus particle. Its technical name is *virion*.

In general, virions of almost all viruses resemble a walnut. A virion has a relatively firm protein shell that contains a piece of genetic material, either RNA or DNA, depending on the type of virus. No known virus contains both RNA and DNA. Some viruses, including the coronaviruses, also are enclosed in a lipid (fatty) envelope.

The virions of all coronaviruses, including SARS-CoV-2, range in size from 80 to 120 nanometers (nm) and have a single piece of RNA inside their shell. To give an idea of the size of SARS-CoV-2 virions, if we could collect all the virions from all the people who have died worldwide from COVID-19 through April 2021, the collection of virions would be almost two-thirds of a cup. That is based on an estimate of 2.9 million people, each with 100 million virions.

Coronaviruses like SARS-CoV-2 have protein protrusions that stick out—little spikes, called *spike proteins*.

Many people believe that the word *corona*—for crown—used in *coronavirus*—comes from the spikes' resemblance to a royal crown. Actually—and here's something you can use to show your friends that you know something about COVID-19—coronaviruses were named for the corona—crown—of the *sun*, during a total eclipse.

I learned this from an article in *Nature*. In 1968, eight virologists announced a new group of viruses with a "characteristic fringe" of projections, an appearance "recalling the *solar corona*"—in other words, the corona of the *sun*.

COVID-19!

The virologists suggested calling the group of viruses *corona-viruses,* "to recall the characteristic appearance by which these viruses are identified in the electron microscope."

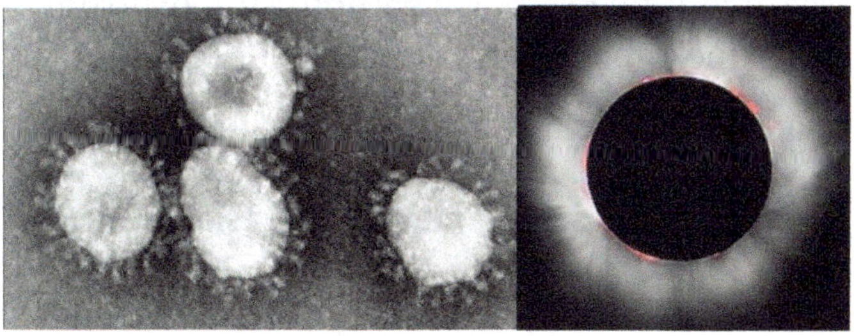

Here's one of the first pictures of the virus,
and a photo of the solar corona during an eclipse.

The spike proteins

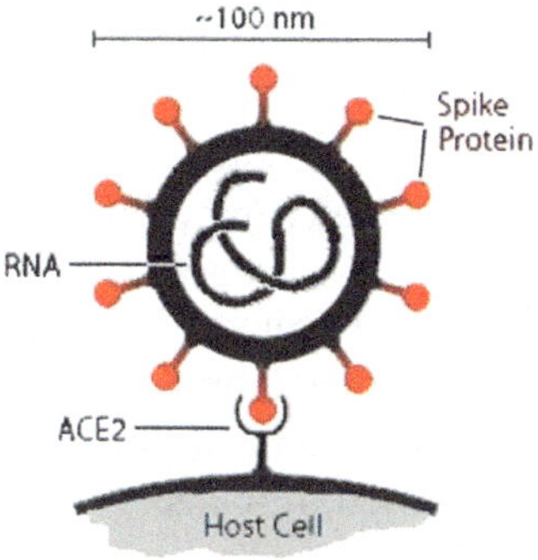

The spikes on some viruses, including SARS-CoV-2, attach the virion to an enzyme protein, called ACE2, on the surface of many host cells (cells the virus can invade). The attachment allows the virion to enter the cell.

The most common host cells are in the lungs, heart, arteries, kidneys, and intestines. These are the typical target organs for SARS-CoV-2 virions and the typical sites of infection. They also have an abundance of ACE2.

Many SARS-CoV-2 vaccines and those under development target the virions' spike protein. The strategy is to block the spike on the virion from being able to attach to the ACE2 enzyme protein on the target cell. If a virion can't attach, it can't infect.

How are viruses different from bacteria?

Viruses are not just small bacteria. A typical bacterial cell contains everything it needs to live without support from other cells. A virus does not. A virus is not a cell.

Let's take a closer look at the differences between the two.

Comparing Viruses and Bacteria

Virus	Bacterial Cell
So small, can't be seen with an optical microscope, but only with an electron microscope	Visible with ordinary optical microscope
A piece of RNA[a] or DNA (never both), enclosed in a protein coat; some viruses have an additional envelope of fatty material	Has DNA as its genetic material and RNA for protein synthesis and for gene regulation
Not "alive," because viruses cannot obtain energy and nutrients to carry out vital functions; do not grow, but are assembled, full size, by an infected cell	Self-sufficient; has its own metabolism, through which it obtains energy from nutrients for its life functions and growth
Reproduction occurs only when a virus takes control of a host cell and "orders" it to make more virus particles like itself	Reproduces by using nutrients to grow larger and divide into two "daughter" cells
Cannot be "killed," but can be inactivated	Can be killed

[a]All coronaviruses contain RNA as their genetic material

Viral Reproduction

During infection, a virion—the infectious form of a virus—enters a living cell. The virion "inserts" its genetic material—RNA or DNA—into the cell, thus taking control of the cell.

The virus's genetic code "instructs" the infected cell to

1) Stop carrying out its normal functions
2) Make more virus particles

The cell releases the newly formed particles, and those virus particles infect more cells.

Each infected cell may produce anywhere from ten to several hundred or even thousands of new virus particles. The time the cell takes to produce the particles may be anywhere from less than an hour to as long as a few days, depending on the type of virus. The typical time for infected cells to release coronaviruses is 12 to 24 hours.

COVID-19!

Is the current virus different from the one that caused SARS?

Yes. SARS-CoV-2, the virus responsible for the current COVID-19 pandemic, is similar to SARS-CoV, the virus that caused the 2003 SARS outbreak, yet the behavior of the new virus, SARS-CoV-2, and our response to it, are very different.

First, the similarities:

- Same size
- Same appearance, viewed with an electron microscope
- Same type of surface spikes
- Same genetic material—RNA rather than DNA
- Same family classification (coronavirus)

The key differences:

- People with COVID-19 shed (release virus when they breathe, cough, or sneeze) SARS-CoV-2 *before* they have symptoms
- People with SARS-CoV start shedding virus only *after* they have symptoms
- SARS-CoV-2 seems to be a far more infectious virus—more likely to spread the infection—than SARS-CoV

Other viruses in the coronavirus family typically infect only one type of animal, such as mice. That animal is called the natural host, in which they cause little or no disease, and rarely infect other animals. When viruses "jump" to a different animal, problems can arise.

It's believed that SARS-CoV-2 originated in bats in China. The bats carrying the virus showed no sign of disease. But SARS-CoV-2 apparently passed from bats to another animal, called an intermediate host. What that animal was isn't known. And then SARS-CoV-2 passed from the intermediate host to humans—an *unnatural host*—and humans developed the disease known as COVID-19.

An alternative explanation for the origin of the virus is that it escaped from the Wuhan Institute of Virology. Although such escapes are possible, and some have happened with other viruses at other research laboratories, it is not known whether SARS-CoV-2 escaped from the Wuhan institute. All information available so far is circumstantial and speculative. Whether any definitive, credible data ever become available remains to be seen. Until then, there can be no definitive answer to the origin of the virus.

About Exposure to the Virus

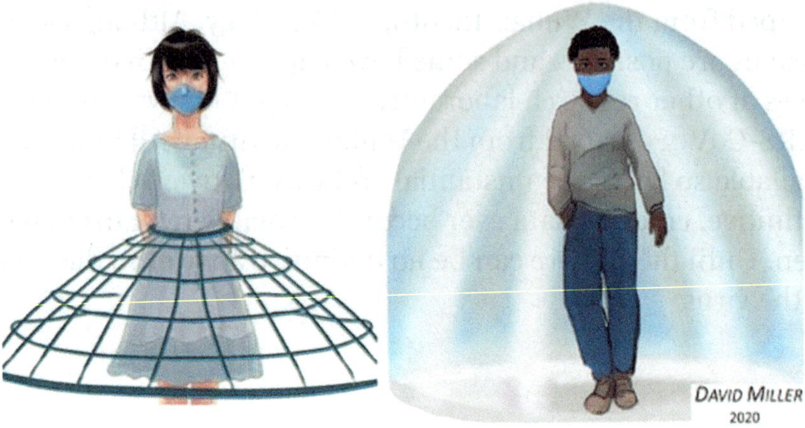

How much exposure do I need to catch COVID-19?

I think what you're asking is, what amount of virus is needed to cause an infection? That's what we call the *infectious dose*. And it varies considerably, depending on the kind of virus.

For example, someone exposed to as few as 10 particles (virions) of influenza virus may come down with influenza. Developing other viral diseases may require exposure to as many as thousands of particles.

No one knows yet how many particles of SARS-CoV-2 are needed to trigger a COVID-19 infection. Clearly, COVID-19 is a highly contagious disease—but *why* is it so contagious?

- For some people, such as the elderly or people with certain health conditions, only a few particles are needed for infection (in other words, the infectious dose is low)
- Some infected people release a lot of virus into their environment, especially just before they develop symptoms

and the first few days of their infection, raising the exposure risk for people around them

A droplet released during a cough or sneeze, or during talking, singing, or shouting, could carry millions of virus particles. A tiny droplet released during calm breathing might not carry many particles—far fewer particles than needed for an infectious dose.

But—

- It's even possible that someone breathing normally could inhale many aerosol droplets during a short period
- If that happens, it's also possible that the number of virus particles accumulating in the nose could exceed the infectious dose

The result: an infection—another case of COVID-19.

****

On a blog he created at the start of the pandemic, Professor Erin Bromage, PhD, of the University of Massachusetts, Dartmouth, estimated that the infectious dose for COVID-19 is 1,000 virions. He based his guess on what is known for influenza virus. His educated guess has not been verified by peer-reviewed data, or by any published data that we're aware of, although several other investigators have reported similar estimates.

Earlier, in 2010, a team headed by Dr. Toru Watanabe published a study suggesting that the infectious dose for SARS-CoV and several other coronaviruses is between 16 and 280 virions, an estimate far lower than Dr. Bromage's. Which estimate is closer to the actual infectious dose for SARS-CoV-2 remains to be seen.

****

COVID-19!

I was within a few feet of a neighbor who came down with COVID-19, and while talking we weren't wearing masks. Does that mean I was exposed to a large amount of virus? And if I catch COVID-19, will I have a worse case?

Close exposure greatly increases the chances that you will become infected—unless you took precautions, such as being vaccinated, wearing your mask, keeping your distance, and washing your hands after talking with your neighbor. These simple precautions improve your chances of avoiding the infection.

But if you *are* infected, will you have a more severe case, because you had a large dose of virus? That's not clear. We just don't know. We don't have the data yet for SARS-CoV-2.

Also, remember that many other factors determine how severe a case of COVID-19 will be. Your immune response is one important factor. If your immune response is insufficient, or delayed, virus levels in your body can become excessively high. On the other hand, if your immune response is too aggressive, severe damage can result. Other health conditions, such as advanced age, diabetes, obesity or overweight, and high blood pressure or other heart or circulatory conditions can contribute to more severe COVID-19 disease.

How is SARS-CoV-2 spread?

Early in the pandemic we knew very little about how the virus spread from person to person. Now that we have much better data, we know that almost all spread is by respiratory droplets or aerosols from infected people.

Early "information" was based either on what seemed to be logical assumptions or on what was known from other viral infections. We now know that contaminated surfaces have rarely, if ever, been a source of spread. Likewise, surfaces of food packages or food within the packages have never been shown to be a source of spread.

Because spread is mainly by respiratory droplets, we now know that masks are far more important than we thought at first. We also know that good ventilation is important for removing contaminated air from interior spaces.

Preventing superspreader events means keeping distance between people (social distancing) and saying "no" to large gatherings, especially indoors. Family gatherings have been a major source of spread, with one infected family member infecting others. But anywhere that people contact other people, without masks, especially where those people are talking, singing, coughing, sneezing, even breathing, a major risk of spread exists. Being *vaccinated, wearing masks, and staying apart from other people are by far the best ways to avoid getting the virus and spreading it to others.*

COVID-19!

Is there any truth to comments on social media, like "Look, it's hardly fatal...see, only 2%."?

We've tried to answer questions in terms that relate to our readers as individuals. People differ in their tolerance for risk, so we'll try to put the fatality (mortality) risk in perspective. Then you can evaluate percentages in terms that relate to you.

Granted, 2% is a small number. But is it really small when it comes to chance of death?

Looking at 2% in terms of odds, it means that 2 of every 100 people will die, or 1 in 50. That's not so low, is it? To put it another way, the Centers for Disease Control and Prevention (CDC) called COVID-19 the third leading cause of death in the U.S. in 2020, behind heart disease and cancer.

Let's look at the data from 2020. First, we need to know the mortality risk from COVID-19, so let's calculate it.

Odds of Dying From COVID-19 in 2020	
Number of U.S. deaths in 2020 that occurred directly or indirectly from COVID-19	A little more than 538,000
Divide that number by the population, 330 million, to get the mortality rate	Mortality rate = 0.16%
Divide 1 by 0.16% to convert to odds	Odds = 1 in 625
Compare some odds:	
Odds of winning the national lottery	1 in 200,000,000
Odds of dying in a plane crash in 2020	1 in 11,000,000
Odds of dying from COVID-19 in 2020	1 in 625

So the mortality rate is 0.16%—even lower—lower by far—than the 2% you quoted. That illustrates how much misinformation there is in social media.

Now let's put those odds of 1 in 625 in perspective.

COVID-19!

The odds of winning a national lottery are about 1 in 200 million. Some states offer better odds: 1 in 6 million. Yet many people aren't bothered by those odds; we've all seen long lines form at lottery ticket windows.

With lotteries, you buy one ticket or a few, and you're out a few bucks, but you have some fun. Your chance of winning, though, is about as close to zero as you can get.

When it comes to your chance of getting COVID-19 and dying from it, your odds are far higher. And if you're in a vulnerable group, such as over 55 years old, or if you have other medical conditions, your odds of dying are higher still.

So get vaccinated, wear your mask, maintain social distance, and follow all other guidelines. No one step is enough; together the recommended steps greatly lower your risk.

If you choose not to follow the guidelines, remember that you're betting your life against highly unfavorable odds.

What are my chances of getting infected, anyway?

The chance that *you,* or any given person, will get COVID-19 depends partly on where you live. Risks are much higher in "hotspots"—*and* in people who aren't taking those *four key precautions: being vaccinated, wearing a mask, social distancing, and handwashing.*

We know—even day-by-day—with reasonable accuracy, the number of confirmed cases of COVID-19 in the U.S. But we don't know the total number of cases—*confirmed plus undiagnosed.*

The reason: many infected people have no symptoms and have not been tested. Obviously, they're not included as confirmed cases.

Estimates are that, for each case of COVID-19 confirmed by testing, *there may be as many as 8 unconfirmed cases.* That's an incredible figure. It's hard to believe.

Here are some other conditions for comparison:

Condition	New cases per 1000 people per year (US)
Diabetes	11
Heart attack	6
COVID-19	4
Breast cancer	2
Prostate cancer	1

As mentioned, the number for COVID-19 in the table is likely too low, because it is based on confirmed cases. Including all infections, whether confirmed or asymptomatic, would increase the number.

COVID-19 is not a disease most people want to have. So, remember those four key guidelines for avoiding infection:

Vaccinating
Masking
Social distancing—at least 6 feet
Handwashing (20 seconds), or use sanitizer

Protecting yourself by following these simple steps, with others mentioned in this book, is most effective if done before you may have been exposed to the virus. Although vaccination is extremely effective at reducing risk of infection, it is not perfect. Vaccinated people can become infected, although their disease is much less severe and their chance of dying is very low.

The importance of combining risk-reducing steps is nicely illustrated by the virologist Ian Mackay, PhD, using an analogy to Swiss cheese, in this article from the New York Times:

https://www.nytimes.com/2020/12/05/health/coronavirus-swiss-cheese-infection-mackay.html

If instead you want to assert your right not to comply with the four guidelines, remember: you are *betting your life and the lives of your family.*

COVID-19!

Some social media posts suggest that the pandemic is a scam and hasn't caused any deaths. What's that all about?

It's not true, of course. The COVID-19 pandemic has caused even more deaths—far more—than the reports indicate.

A single underlying cause of death is listed on death certificates. Although listing up to 20 additional causes is permitted, almost 60 percent of death certificates list only one or two causes.

That can be misleading. Often several medical problems are present and may have contributed to death. Some may even have been the true cause, instead of the cause listed. But the *number* of death certificates provides a reliable death count.

Let's look at CDC data for normal years, such as 2015 through 2019, the five years before the first year of the pandemic.

The chart shows total deaths per week for each of those five years.

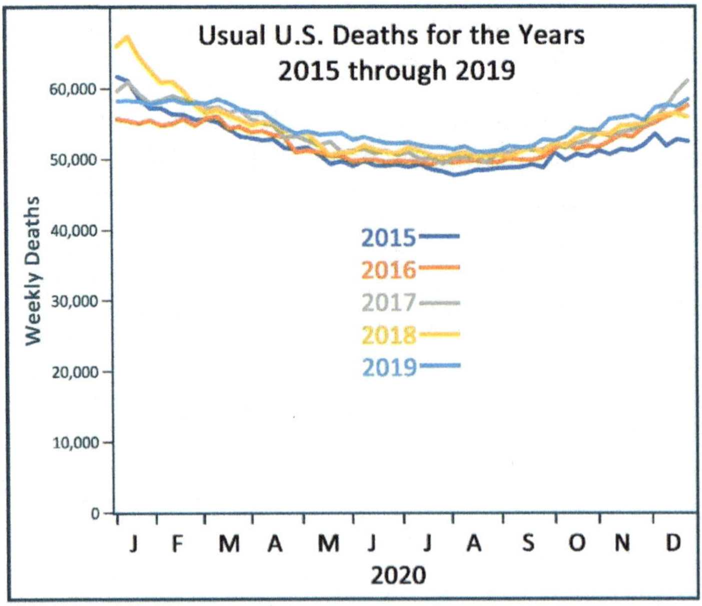

Amazing how similar the lines are.

The chart shows several interesting things.

✓The number of U.S. deaths is reproducible and predictable from one year to the next, unless a major catastrophe occurs. That didn't happen in those five years.

✓Deaths increased during winter months, probably because of increases in the number of seasonal conditions, such as influenza and other respiratory diseases, and suicides (winter depression; severe "winter blues").

✓Weekly deaths increased as the population increased in all months from 2015 to 2019.

Now let's compare those five years with the pandemic year 2020. The chart below shows weekly data from Johns Hopkins University.

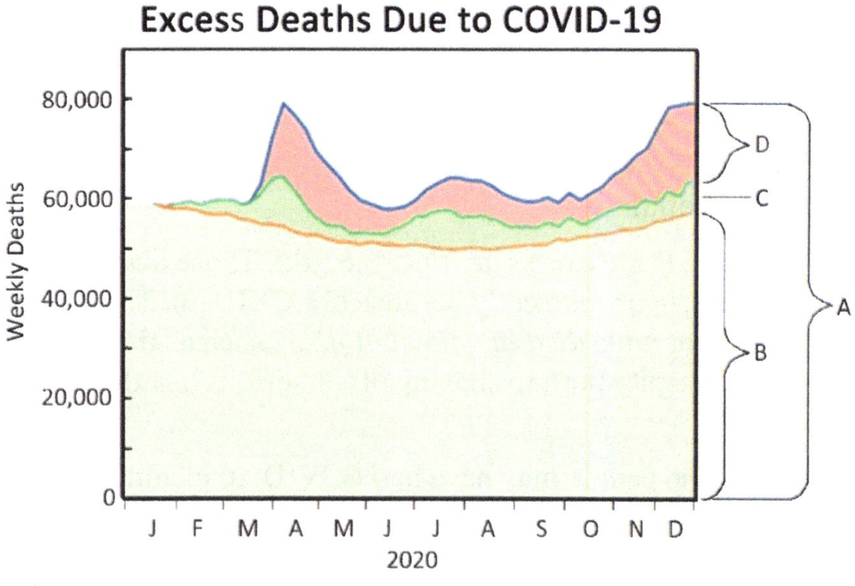

A: Total deaths from all causes, 2020
B: Average of deaths from all causes, 2015 to 2019
C: Deaths recorded as due to COVID-19 = 333,258
D: Deaths indirectly due to COVID-19 = 205,124
C + D = 538,382 excess deaths due to COVID-19

Bracket A shows all deaths, regardless of cause, during the pandemic year, 2020: 3,318,255. This number is reliable because it's a count of all filed death certificates.

Bracket B is the average of yearly deaths during the previous, non-pandemic five years: 2,779,873. These deaths would have been expected whether or not we'd had a pandemic. This number, too, is reliable, because it's based on counts of death certificates.

Bracket C is all deaths reported to CDC in 2020 as caused by COVID-19: 333,258 deaths. This number is not firm. What is recorded as the primary cause of death often is a matter of opinion rather than being based on hard data, such as a test result positive for SARS-CoV-2.

Bracket D is all deaths caused *indirectly* by COVID-19: 205,124. Although not recorded as *due to* COVID-19, many of those deaths occurred because people were unable or unwilling to seek medical care for problems such as heart conditions, advanced diabetes, or high blood pressure. This number, too, isn't firm. It depends on a physician's judgment—choosing a patient's primary cause of death from what often is a complex set of medical conditions.

Brackets C + D are *excess deaths:* 538,382. Those deaths occurred *directly* or *indirectly* because of COVID-19. Those people *would not have died in a normal year*, such as the previous five years, despite perhaps having other serious health conditions.

Some of these people may have had COVID-19 in addition to their other conditions, but their death certificates did not state COVID-19 as the primary cause of death (that is, they were not reported to CDC as COVID-19 deaths). This number is firm, because it is based on the number of death certificates. But the distribution of deaths between brackets C and D may not be firm.

COVID-19!

In the excess deaths group (deaths unattributed to a specific cause, bracket C + D) COVID-19 may have been the *direct* or *indirect* cause of death, or the decedent may not have had COVID-19:

✓COVID-19 patients could have died from a heart attack or stroke unrelated to their infection, or from suicide that wouldn't have occurred in a normal year

✓Or, COVID-19 patients could have died from a heart attack that wasn't adequately treated, because hospitals had no room for timely admission

✓Or, postponement of cancer screenings, to avoid COVID-19 exposure, may have led to death from an undetected malady

✓Or, local political pressure may have caused an under-recording of COVID-19 deaths; if so, the deaths not recorded as due to COVID-19 would show up in D instead of C

The pandemic has *reduced* the number of deaths related to car-driving. Fewer car crashes have occurred, because of lockdowns and stay-at-home orders. Air pollution is greatly reduced, with fewer pollution-related deaths. If car-driving hadn't been reduced, the blue curve would be a little higher, but we don't know exactly how much because we don't have the data.

This analysis shows that the damage caused by COVID-19 in 2020 was much worse than the official numbers indicate. We had 538,382 deaths resulting directly and indirectly from COVID-19. That's almost twice the reported number, 333,258

What are the symptoms of COVID-19?

The CDC keeps a symptom list and updates it periodically.

https://www.cdc.gov/coronavirus/2019-ncov/symptoms-testing/symptoms.html

Symptoms of COVID-19 may be mild to severe. They appear 2 to 14 days (the incubation period) after the infected person is exposed to the virus. In December 2020, the CDC listed the following symptoms, noting that not all possible symptoms are included:

- Fever or chills
- Cough
- Shortness of breath or difficulty breathing
- Fatigue
- Muscle or body aches
- Headache
- New loss of sense of taste or smell
- Sore throat
- Congestion or runny nose
- Nausea or vomiting
- Diarrhea

According to a publication of the County of Los Angeles Public Health, many of the symptoms are common to other respiratory or viral illnesses, but "new loss of smell or taste appears to be more specific to COVID-19."

http://publichealth.lacounty.gov/acd/ncorona2019/clinicaldx/

And another recent publication adds dizziness to the symptoms list. The dizziness, also called vertigo, can be so severe that the person may have trouble standing without falling.

Is there a way to tell if someone who may have COVID-19 needs emergency help?

Yes. CDC lists the following emergency warning signs, and adds that if anyone is showing any of the signs, **seek emergency medical care immediately.**

The signs:

- Trouble breathing
- Persistent pain or pressure in the chest
- New confusion
- Inability to wake or stay awake
- Bluish lips or face

Call 911 or call ahead to your local emergency facility: Notify the operator that you are seeking care for someone who has or may have COVID-19.

My cousin is visiting us, and he's been having some nausea and diarrhea. Could he have COVID-19?

It's possible. About a third of patients develop intestinal problems—loss of appetite, nausea, vomiting, abdominal pain, and diarrhea—as part of their COVID-19 illness. Sometimes intestinal problems are the first sign a person notices. Because of the possibility that your cousin has COVID-19, he should quarantine for 10 days.

Infectious virus has been isolated from stools of infected patients and from the intestinal linings of patients who died from the disease. In fact, the virus can be isolated from stool even several weeks after the illness has cleared up and after viral tests using nasal swabs detect no virus.

Surveys have shown that two out of three patients who had positive test results for intestinal virus didn't develop any gastrointestinal symptoms. Fecal material could be a source of the virus and a means of transmission.

Urine specimens do not contain SARS-CoV-2.

I have a slight fever, and I'm getting a dry cough. I'm worried that I might have COVID-19. What should I do?

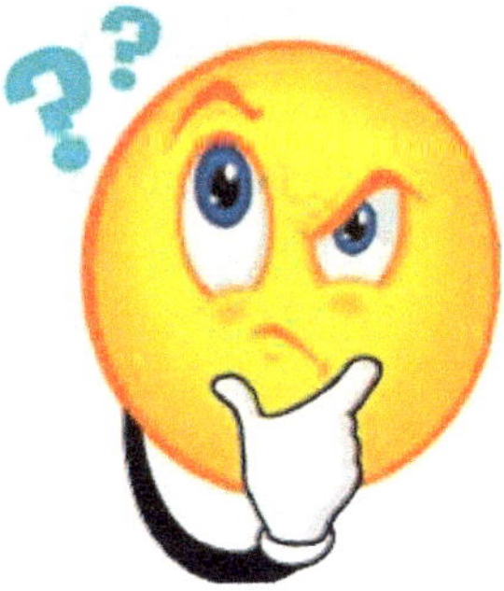

Call your doctor if you've been exposed to someone with COVID-19, or think you've been exposed, and have any of the following:

≈ A fever

≈ A cough, or difficulty breathing

≈ Loss of your sense of smell or taste

Be sure to call before you go to your doctor's office or to an emergency department.

There are two reasons for calling:

- Maybe a visit isn't necessary; the doctor or the doctor's office might be able to help you over the phone
- The doctor might want you to wait outside or in your car until an examining room is ready, so you don't expose other people—or yourself—more than is necessary

Your doctor can tell you more about whether you should be tested, how to get tested, and how to seek medical treatment while lowering the risk of infecting others.

I've been having some symptoms, and my doctor is arranging a COVID-19 test for me. What do I need to know?

There are two kinds of tests: diagnostic tests, to see if you *have* the disease right now; and antibody tests, to see if you recently *had* the disease. Antibodies are special proteins that your body makes to defend against infectious agents such as viruses. The antibodies react with and inactivate an antigen, which is a part of a virus or other invader.

You'll probably have one of the two kinds of diagnostic tests: a molecular test or an antigen test.

COVID-19 Tests Answer Your Questions

"Do I have COVID-19 now?" ⟶ A DIAGNOSTIC TEST
A Molecular Test (for viral RNA)
OR
An Antigen Test (for viral protein)

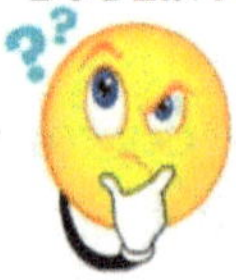

"Did I recently have COVID-19?" ⟶ AN ANTIBODY TEST

Molecular tests detect viral RNA; antigen tests detect viral protein. If RNA or the viral protein is present, you are currently infected with SARS-CoV-2.

Something you need to know (although you've heard this before!): What I'm going to tell you about these tests is accurate now, but things are changing very quickly. We're going to update our information as often as we can on our website (www.covid-19faqbook.com) and in new editions of this book.

Another point: No test is 100% accurate. Your doctor is having you tested apparently because your symptoms suggest you may have COVID-19. Your doctor's impression of your current clinical condition may be every bit as important as your test results.

If your swab test result is positive—it says you have COVID-19—that's good evidence. You can accept that.

But what if you have a negative test result?

Well, that's where your doctor's judgment comes in, as I mentioned before. Even with a negative test result, if your symptoms strongly suggest COVID-19, your doctor probably will want you to self-isolate anyway and perhaps will want to test you again.

This table summarizes the tests that tell whether or not you are infected (diagnosis) by testing for viral RNA. Keep in mind that new tests are being developed, and some are already being marketed.

Diagnostic Tests for SARS-CoV-2: Molecular (for Viral RNA)		
Three types of test procedures for viral RNA	Real Time-Polymerase chain reaction test (RT-PCR) Nucleic acid amplification test (NAAT) Loop-mediated isothermal amplification test (LAMP)	
Sample obtained from	Back of the mouth Oropharyngeal swab (OP)	Back of the nose Nasopharyngeal swab (NP)
Sampling procedure	OP: Swab is inserted through the mouth to the back of the throat and rotated to collect secretions	NP: Swab is inserted deep into the nasal cavity and rotated to collect secretions
Laboratory procedure	Mucus sample is tested for SARS- CoV-2 RNA	
Diagnosis	Active COVID-19	
Comments	Patient acceptance is more likely with the OP than with the NP swab	Some patients find the NP procedure uncomfortable
	The RT-PCR, NAAT, and LAMP tests are usually highly accurate	

Another approach is to determine whether or not you're infected by testing for viral protein, the antigen. Here's a table summarizing antigen tests.

Diagnostic Test for SARS-CoV-2: Antigen (for Viral Protein)	
Test name	Rapid Diagnostic Antigen Test
Name of swab (by location)	Oropharyngeal swab (OP), or nasopharyngeal swab (NP)
Sampling procedure	Swab is inserted deep through the mouth or nose to the back of the throat and rotated to collect secretions
Laboratory procedure	Mucus sample is tested for SARS- CoV-2 antigen (protein)
Diagnosis	Active COVID-19
Comments	Results are available much sooner than with a PCR test, but the test is not as likely as the PCR test to diagnose early infections Positive test results usually are highly accurate; negative test results may require confirmation with a PCR test

Both types of diagnostic tests use samples from the nose or throat. Those samples contain virus during active infection. Some people don't mind the nasal swabs; others do. You can ask if the oropharyngeal procedure—the OP procedure—is available. Some people prefer it.

So those are the diagnostic tests. The other type of test is an antibody test, to find out if you've already had COVID-19. The table below summarizes the antibody test.

Antibody Test	
Purpose	Results indicate if there's been a previous infection (at least one to two weeks ago) with SARS-CoV-2; a positive result shows that the patient had COVID-19
Other names	Serological test, blood test
Specimen collection	Fingerstick or blood draw
Diagnostic procedure	Check for antibody against SARS-CoV-2
Diagnosis	+ Positive test result shows that the patient *most likely has had* an infection with SARS-CoV-2 - Negative test result *suggests* that the patient *hasn't* been infected (*hasn't* had SARS-CoV-2); it may be necessary to repeat the antibody test

Note that, if you have a positive test result, your doctor will almost certainly accept that as meaning that you did, in fact, recently have COVID-19.

A negative test result, well, that's suggestive; it suggests you haven't had COVID-19 but doesn't rule out the possibility. It can also mean you've had the test too soon after your infection, because it takes several weeks for your body to make antibodies.

As for how long you'll have to wait for the results, the office where you took the tests can tell you when they expect to send them out.

Time Required for Test Results	
Molecular Diagnostic Test	Same day (some areas), to up to one week
Antigen Diagnostic Test	One hour or less
Antibody Test	Same day (some areas), to up to one week

Remember, though, that the time required isn't just for doing the test. The laboratory may get backed up preparing the result and doing the paperwork.

Newly available tests

At-home collection tests are available, some without prescription. For some tests, the patient provides a sample, such as placing some saliva in a tube included in the test kit, and sends the sample to the laboratory for analysis. Patients themselves perform other tests, with results available within a half hour or so. These tests are in early stages of development or deployment, so not much is known about their accuracy and usefulness.

Rapid, point-of-care diagnostic tests

These rapid tests can be molecular tests or antigen tests. If your doctor orders a rapid diagnostic test, a technician in the doctor's office will collect a sample from your nose or throat, and the sample will be analyzed right there, in the doctor's office. In just minutes, everyone has the answer as to whether you have COVID-19 or not.

Vaccines

GET YOUR *VACCINATION!*

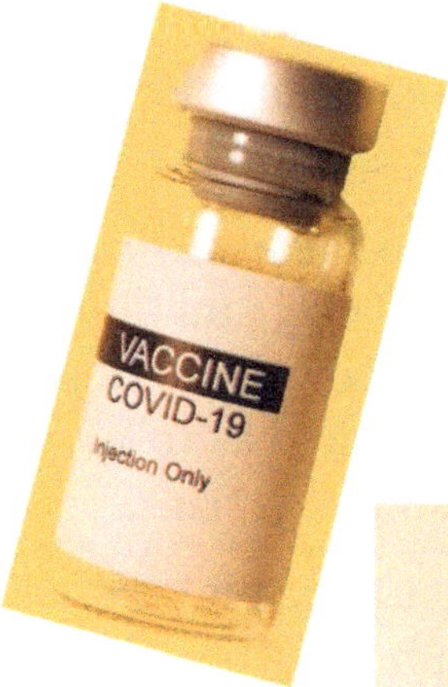

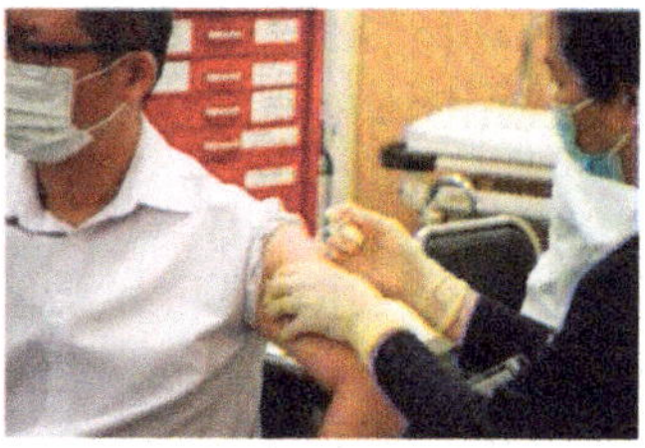

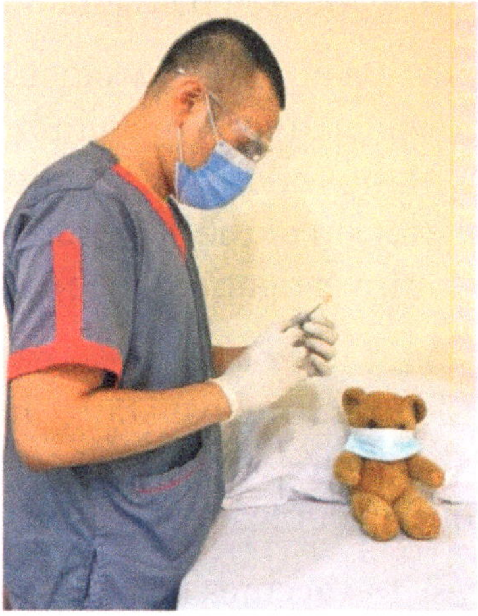

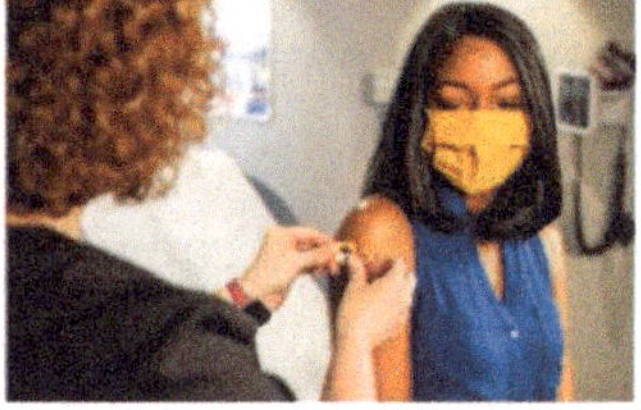

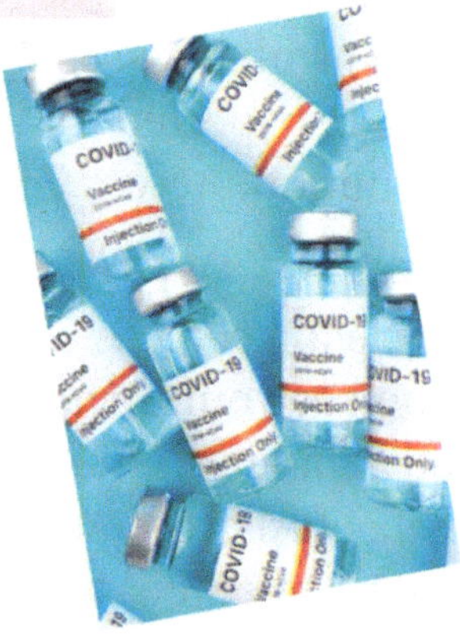

COVID-19!

Should I get vaccinated?

Almost certainly you should—many good reasons say *get vaccinated*, and no reasons say not to. The two exceptions: the CDC advises against getting the COVID-19 vaccine if you've had a severe allergic reaction to any of the ingredients in the current vaccines. And if you've had a severe allergic reaction to other types of vaccines, or to certain injected medications, be sure to ask your health care provider if the vaccine is right for you.

As of this writing (May 2021), three vaccines are available in the U.S.: the Pfizer-BioNTech, for ages 16 and above; and the Moderna and Johnson & Johnson vaccines, both for ages 18 and above. The age for eligibility is being lowered as results from clinical trials are evaluated by regulatory agencies.

Clinical trials have shown all three vaccines to be highly effective for decreasing serious illness, hospitalization, and deaths due to COVID-19, with no reports of significant safety issues (except that administration of the Johnson & Johnson vaccine was paused briefly for investigation of a possible safety issue).

As vaccine supplies built up, vaccines were given according to individual state guidelines. In most states, health care workers on the front lines taking care of COVID-19 patients were top priority. Healthy young people have been lower priority.

At this writing, access to vaccines has become easier. Production of available vaccines continues to increase, and new vaccines are expected to finish trials in 2021 and be authorized for distribution. Access is being extended to lower-priority groups, including school-age children.

Be sure to keep up to date in your state so you can get your shot as soon as your turn comes up. Once vaccinated, you'll be in good company. Dr. Anthony Fauci, director of the National Institute of Allergy and Infectious Diseases, received his second dose in December 2020, and four former presidents have been vaccinated.

COVID-19!

What about the new technology, mRNA—is it safe?

This question came from my wife, Barbara, when vaccines became available. Because I thought using mRNA was a new technology, I wanted to learn more about it before deciding to be vaccinated. What I found was:

- Although the Pfizer/BioNTech and Moderna vaccines for COVID-19 are new, in that they became available very recently, they are actually the result of about 25 years of development
- A turning point in 2005 that made the vaccine possible was a clever and scientifically creative discovery of how to make the mRNA more stable (in my opinion that work by Drs. Katalin Kariko and Drew Weissman merits a Nobel Prize; see below)
- The mRNA in the vaccine codes for only a part of the spike protein, not whole virus, so it is biologically impossible for the mRNA to cause a cell to start making viruses—in other words, the vaccine can't cause COVID-19
- It is also biologically impossible for the mRNA in the vaccine to change a person's DNA
- There is no possibility that the vaccine can cause a person to lose fertility or to have a miscarriage
- Biologically, the mRNA itself is very unlikely to cause side effects, although it's possible that the delivery system could—the delivery system being the shells (actually, tiny bags formed of a fatty membrane than enclose the mRNA) used by the Pfizer/BioNTech and Moderna vaccines, or the adenovirus shell used by the Johnson & Johnson vaccine

- The clinical trials of the vaccines showed them to be highly effective, much more so than vaccines for other viral diseases, and to have no significant side effects

All of this information reassured me that the vaccines were quite safe and effective, so my wife and I received the two doses of Pfizer COVID-19 vaccine as soon as we could schedule them.

****

Katalin ("Kati") Kariko, PhD, endured long years of obscurity as she struggled to obtain grants or funds to carry out her work. Prevailing wisdom was that Dr. Kariko's ideas about using messenger RNA (mRNA) to "instruct" human cells to make proteins they would not ordinarily make was, well, outlandish—so outlandish that her ideas didn't merit the customary funding or grants. Another possible source of support was venture money, but venture capitalists weren't interested in supporting her work. So without funding, Dr. Kariko was demoted academically.

But she persisted.

In 1997 she teamed up with Drew Weissman, MD, PhD, an immunologist. In 2005, they made a key discovery: a modification of the mRNA so that it was not rejected by the immune system. That discovery made it possible for the mRNA that previously had worked only in cultured cells (which have no immune system)—to work in people as well.

That stroke of scientific creativity transformed vaccine development. And it became the basis for the life-saving mRNA vaccines.

Procedures that previously took many years now required just a few months. The key: the entirely synthetic mRNA, which can be made to order based on the genetic sequence of the desired protein. With it, vast amounts of vaccine could be produced much more easily and quickly. No longer was it necessary to spend the many months of tinkering with quirky biological problems that conventional vaccines require.

Any concerns about safety are ill-founded. Because the genetic code embedded in synthetic mRNA is not found in nature, the vaccine cannot modify any of the body's normal functions. All it can do is work like a new recipe telling the body's cells how to make the spike protein. And the spike protein "teaches" the body's immune system to make antibodies—stopping the virus from causing infection.

Over time, we'll see many other applications of this new technology. And many people will thank the creative woman who brought the new technology into fruition, Dr. Katalin Kariko. The woman so many ignored for so long.

What other vaccines are available?

At the time of this writing, other vaccines are either just becoming available or are in late trial stage. We don't have enough information on these new vaccines to be able to make any statements about them. We plan to post questions and answers as in this book on our website (www.covid-19faqbook.com) as new reliable information comes out. Those questions and answers will be incorporated in a second edition of this book to be published when justified by the new information.

COVID-19!

I'm worried that the vaccine makers may have cut corners. I hear it usually takes 10 or so years to develop a vaccine, and these three vaccines didn't take even a year! How did that happen?

Operation Warp Speed gets most of the credit. On May 15, 2020, the White House announced Operation Warp Speed to expedite the development, production, and distribution of COVID-19 vaccines, therapeutics, and diagnostics. The goal was to produce and deliver 300 million doses of safe, effective vaccines, with initial doses to be available by January 2021. Thus, it was the federal government, not the pharmaceutical companies, that took most of the financial risk. And the companies would benefit if their vaccine was safe and effective, giving them incentives to succeed.

Vaccine development, like all drug development, requires huge capital investments, and it entails financial risks that can quickly throw a company into bankruptcy. A vaccine that looks promising in one stage of development can fail the next.

Therefore, companies that risk involvement in such enterprises typically proceed slowly and carefully, making sure the current step is okay before investing in the next, usually far more expensive step. With the federal government, not the companies, taking the financial risk, many companies charged ahead. Vaccine manufacture started even before trials were over. If a trial failed—if the vaccine was ineffective—the government, not the pharmaceutical company, lost the bet.

Another important reason for Operation Warp Speed's success was mRNA technology—an approach developed over the past 25 years and already perfected during vaccine development efforts for other viral diseases. This relatively new approach is much faster than older methods, and its safety had already been tested when it was used to develop other vaccines. Moreover, the approach allows scientists to quickly alter a vaccine if variants of the target virus were to arise—as, in fact, they already have.

To infect, SARS-CoV-2 attaches to the cell using the spike protein. The coronaviruses we know of in the SARS-CoV-2 group have very similar spike proteins, and those spike proteins are exposed on the surface of the virion, where antibodies can easily attach. So it was clear to vaccine designers what their target would be and how to attack it. In fact, the location and susceptibility of the targets—the spike proteins—made it easier to design a vaccine for SARS-CoV-2 than for many other kinds of virus.

Still another factor contributing to the extraordinarily rapid vaccine development was ease in recruiting participants for clinical trials. Recruitment usually proceeds slowly because the pool of potential participants is limited. But when recruitment for the COVID-19 vaccine began, only a small percentage of the U.S. population had been infected with the coronavirus. So people—20,000 to 30,000 of them—quickly came forth, eager for a chance to be protected against COVID-19.

COVID-19!

I've had two doses of the Pfizer vaccine, the second dose three weeks ago. What can I do now? Can I fly, for example?

Here's the CDC's advice, as of March 9, 2021. Keep in mind this advice could change quickly—in our experience, that can be a day or two—so check our website for possible updates.

First, a definition. The CDC considers people fully vaccinated:

- 2 weeks after their second dose in a 2-dose series, like the Pfizer or Moderna vaccines, or
- 2 weeks after a single-dose vaccine, like Johnson & Johnson's Janssen vaccine

If it has been less than 2 weeks since your injection, or if you still need your second dose, you are not fully protected. Continue taking preventive steps.

After you're fully vaccinated

Being fully vaccinated tremendously lowers your risk of infection, but does not eliminate the risk—your chance of being infected does not go to zero. So your actions after being vaccinated depend on your tolerance for risk.

If you want to be extra cautious, continue taking precautions in public places: wearing a mask, staying six feet from others, avoiding crowds and poorly ventilated areas, and washing hands for 20 seconds.

- You can gather indoors with fully vaccinated people without wearing a mask.
- You can gather indoors with unvaccinated people from one other household (for example, visiting with relatives who all live together) without masks, unless any of those people or anyone they live with has an increased risk for severe illness from COVID-19.

- If you've been around someone who has COVID-19, you do not need to stay away from others or get tested unless you have symptoms.
  - However, if you live in a group setting (like a correctional or detention facility or group home) and are around someone who has COVID-19, you should still stay away from others for 14 days and get tested, even if you don't have symptoms.

For now, if you've been fully vaccinated:

- You should still take steps to protect yourself and others in many situations, like wearing a mask, staying at least 6 feet apart from others, and avoiding crowds and poorly ventilated spaces. Take these precautions whenever you are:
  - In public
  - Gathering with unvaccinated people from more than one other household
  - Visiting with an unvaccinated person who is at increased risk of severe illness or death from COVID-19 or who lives with a person at increased risk
- You should still avoid medium or large-sized gatherings.
- You should still delay domestic and international travel. If you do travel, you'll still need to follow CDC requirements and recommendations in effect when you fly.
- You should still watch out for symptoms of COVID-19, especially if you've been around someone who is sick. If you have symptoms of COVID-19, you should get tested and stay home and away from others.
- You will still need to follow guidance at your workplace.

COVID-19!

Sorry, my friend, about your desire to fly—as you can see, delaying domestic and international travel is still recommended—but those two little words, “for now,” at least give us some hope that we can be in the air again before too long.

So, these are the basics about what you can and cannot do after vaccination. For details, go to the CDC website:

https://www.cdc.gov/coronavirus/2019-ncov/vaccines.

And remember to check our website as well.

I've already had COVID-19. Should I be vaccinated? And if so, when?

Yes, you should be vaccinated even if you've had COVID-19, because we don't know how long protection lasts. There aren't enough data yet showing how long people are protected from getting sick again after they've recovered from COVID-19.

It's even possible that you could get COVID-19 again; although we know that happens, data do not support the view of many people that reinfection is common.

One additional thought: if you were treated for COVID-19 with monoclonal antibodies or convalescent plasma, you should wait 90 days before getting a COVID-19 vaccine. If you're not sure what treatments you had, talk with your health care professional.

I thought I couldn't have vaccines, because I'm immunosuppressed. So why am I supposed to get the COVID-19 vaccine?

That's a great question—and you're right; people who are immunosuppressed can't have the measles, mumps, and rubella (MMR) vaccines, for example.

But—and it's a big *but*—those are *live* vaccines. They contain small amounts of active but very weakened viruses.

The COVID-19 vaccines from Pfizer and Moderna don't contain any active viruses. Those vaccines work by instructing your own cells to make viral spike protein (but no other parts of the virus) and your immune system "learns" how to block the virus from infecting.

So both vaccines are safe for immunosuppressed people, *except* of course people who are severely allergic to ingredients in the vaccine.

I've heard that vaccines are important in keeping variants away. Can you explain how?

Yes, that is important. Variants occur due to virus replication—the more the virus replicates, the greater the chance for variants.

It's because each time an infected cell makes new viral RNA, there is a high chance of a mutation. Mutations are mistakes in the genetic code embedded in the RNA.

Most mutations are meaningless, but sometimes a group of mutations creates a variant with new properties.

Some new variants are less infectious and die out. But if the new properties increase the virus's ability to infect, or the mutations in the variant cause the cell to make more new particles than it would make with the original virus, the variant can spread more easily and be more deadly.

New variants may also be resistant to vaccines, so that vaccines now in use may no longer be effective at preventing infection and disease.

The ability to quickly modify a vaccine to be effective against new variants is an extremely important feature of the new mRNA vaccines (Pfizer/BioNTech and Moderna).

Getting your vaccination is important in protecting you but it also helps prevent new, and potentially more deadly, variants from occurring.

About Immunity and the Pandemic

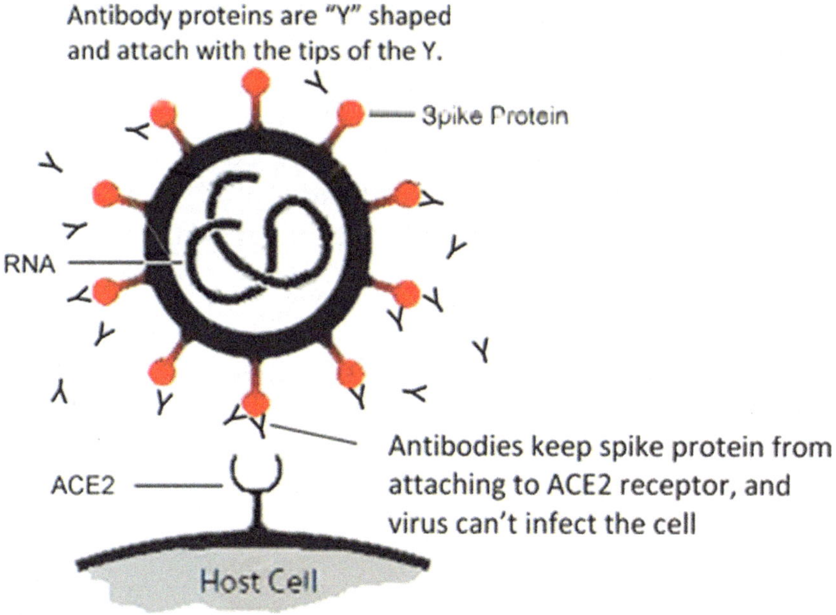

How do people become immune?

People can develop immunity in either of two ways:

– By being vaccinated

– By having the disease *and* developing antibodies as a result

There's a lot we don't know yet about COVID-19. We don't know if everyone who has the disease develops antibodies, and, if antibodies do develop, how long they last. Nor do we know if someone who survives COVID-19 becomes immune as a result. We do know that, with the coronaviruses that cause the common cold, immunity lasts only about three months to possibly up to a year, in some cases.

Nor do we know how long protection from a COVID-19 vaccination will last. Eventually the answer will come from clinical trials—*if* the participants are followed for at least several months—and *if* participants' antibody levels are measured periodically.

The answer could also come by testing people for a period of time after they've been vaccinated.

It is also possible that infection with some other virus, not necessarily one related to SARS-CoV-2, could give at least partial protection against SARS-CoV-2.

Such partial protection (called a cross-reaction) is known to occur in some viral infections. It's possible that some cases of COVID-19 have been milder than they might have been, because of the patients' previous viral infections.

Someone said that the way we're going, most people will become infected, and then COVID-19 will just die out. Is that possible?

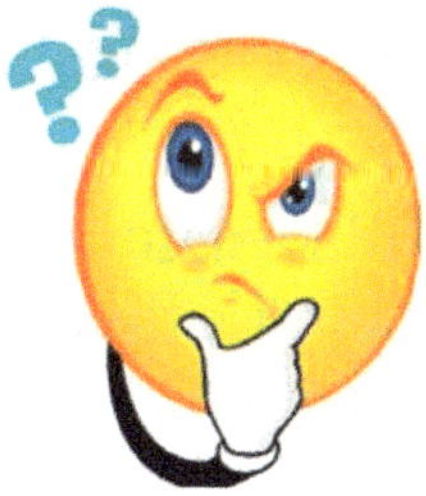

That's almost certainly not possible. What you're describing is herd immunity. When enough people in a community have been infected and have become immune, we say that herd immunity has developed. Obviously, once that happens, it's more difficult for the virus to find susceptible people to infect.

Herd immunity from natural infection has never happened, however. Smallpox was widespread for thousands of years with high rates of infection and mortality, yet herd immunity did not occur. Vaccination eventually stopped smallpox infections.

As scientists at Johns Hopkins explain herd immunity: "For example, if 80% of a population is immune to a virus, four out of every five people who encounter someone with the disease won't get sick (and won't spread the disease any further)."

They estimate that usually "70% to 90% of a population needs immunity to achieve herd immunity." They think that, with the current coronavirus, at least 70% of the population will need to be immune if we're to have herd immunity.

To use the U.S. as an example, with its population of 330 million people, 231 million cases would have to occur to achieve a 70% case rate. A 1% case fatality rate means that over 2 million people would have to die to achieve herd immunity—and those numbers are on the optimistic side. And even after sacrificing all those people, herd immunity from natural infection would probably not occur and the pandemic would continue.

Herd immunity can and does occur by vaccination, and that is quite possible with the new vaccines, if enough people get vaccinated.

When—and how—will this pandemic end? Only through herd immunity?

No one knows when, but we do know several ways the pandemic might end. The first three ways involve herd immunity.

1. The current vaccines—and perhaps new ones as well—become widely accepted and used. Unlike natural infections, vaccines can provide herd immunity, because they can be administered to a large segment of the population. Widespread infections don't need to occur.

A vaccine could save many lives that would be lost if the pandemic were to run its course. FDA gave emergency use authorization (EUA) for two vaccines at the end of 2020, and FDA expects to grant several more EUAs for vaccines in 2021.

Dr. Edward Jenner developed a vaccine in 1796 to prevent smallpox, which was widespread worldwide and had not been stopped by natural herd immunity. Because of vaccination, no smallpox outbreaks have occurred in the U.S. since 1949. According to the World Health Assembly, smallpox was eliminated worldwide in 1980, which allowed smallpox vaccinations to be stopped throughout the world in that year. A polio vaccine has almost eradicated polio worldwide; eradication could occur if opposition to vaccination were to end. Unfounded opposition to vaccines in general, which seems to be increasing because of misinformation in social media, could prevent sufficient vaccinations to provide herd immunity, and the pandemic and deaths could continue.

2. Herd immunity develops naturally. In this scenario, the pandemic continues to infect people across the globe. When a high enough percentage of the population has been infected, the pandemic ends. It ends because there aren't enough susceptible people left—people who could become infected—to keep it going. In this case we could say that herd immunity has ended the pandemic.

It's not necessary for everyone to be infected for herd immunity to occur. With measles, for example, herd immunity could occur with 95% of the population infected. With SARS-CoV-2, it is about 70%. *The bad news is that herd immunity by natural infection rarely, if ever, stops an epidemic or pandemic.* The influenza pandemic of 1918 to 1920, for example, infected only about a third of the world's population, which is not high enough for herd immunity to occur. Letting a pandemic rip through a population *does not work and needlessly kills many people.* Sweden tried to stop the current pandemic by allowing gatherings without masks or social distancing, and the country has paid the price in one of the highest mortality rates while the pandemic continues to rage there.

3. A carefully controlled spread of infection allows herd immunity to develop. Some countries are considering temporarily lifting the requirement for social distancing and mask wearing for COVID-19, especially for younger people, who are less likely to have serious disease. Officials believe doing so would allow the virus to spread for a short time. If the officials managed this scenario carefully, the number of people infected could be controlled. Herd immunity would build up, eventually stopping the spread.

The key to doing this without overwhelming hospitals and other resources is by carefully adjusting the timing. The social distancing requirement would need to be eased gradually and the population would have to be cooperative. With proper timing, hospitals would not be overwhelmed, and deaths would be minimized. Again, this assumes that infection provides solid immunity—and that's far from certain.

Countries that have tried allowing natural infections to occur have found that many people have died needlessly. Achieving herd immunity by natural infection *should not be tried—it has never worked.*

4. Intensive use of non-pharmaceutical approaches. By extreme enforcement of lockdowns in various cities, China brought its pandemic under control. Its economy recovered, even without a vaccine. Other countries have also succeeded in stopping the pandemic within their borders with non-pharmaceutical means. Having a vaccine isn't essential for stopping an epidemic or pandemic, but it requires a strong, decisive government and a cooperative population.

5. An effective antiviral drug is developed. For example, more than two dozen drugs are now available to treat HIV, and these medications have brought the HIV/AIDS pandemic under control. Yet no vaccine for HIV/AIDS has been developed, despite extensive effort and many clinical trials. Many drugs are being looked at as possible treatments for COVID-19.

Results of a large, well-designed clinical trial of remdesivir were published in November 2020. Although remdesivir treatment shortened the length of hospitalization and decreased the need for ventilation for the patients that received the drug, the effects were modest. Nevertheless, remdesivir remains the only drug that treats the viral infection. Other treatments provide support and decrease symptoms.

Chloroquine and hydroxychloroquine have been discussed, but both carry significant toxicities—especially for patients whose age or health conditions puts them at highest risk. Moreover, results published in early May 2020 and reports from more thorough trials since then have shown convincingly that neither drug is effective in treating COVID-19.

Bringing to market an effective drug that treats the viral infection robustly will take time. All drugs are carefully tested before winning the approval of the Food and Drug Administration (FDA), and FDA requires extensive testing to ensure that the drug is safe and effective.

What happens if I'm exposed to the virus?

Your response depends on how much virus you're exposed to. You may not even be aware of a small exposure. A larger exposure may lead to an infection, perhaps even a severe infection.

Let's say you breathe in two or three aerosol droplets, and let's say each contains 10 virus particles. Even if the virus particles infect a few cells in your respiratory tract, your body has some simple defenses to keep that small infection from spreading through your body.

But what if you receive a much larger amount of virus? Suppose someone near you sneezes or coughs, releasing big droplets that contain several thousand, or even a million active virus particles? That's far more than the threshold number for infection, called the *infectious dose* (which is probably somewhere around 500 virus particles for SARS-CoV-2). Our simple, first line of defense can't manage such an exposure and early infection.

So then your full immune system revs up. It starts making antibodies. Those are protein molecules that are specific—meaning they attach to only one target protein. And those antibodies can bring the infection under control.

How do they do it?

Take a look at the diagram at the beginning of this section. The antibodies go after proteins on the surface of the virus (SARS-CoV-2). Some of those antibodies target the spike protein. They attach to the spike, blocking the virus from infecting cells in the respiratory tract.

But for two or so weeks, until there are enough antibodies to stop the virus, the virus can spread throughout the lungs and other parts of the body, causing the disease called COVID-19.

I'm immunosuppressed—will that change my response if I'm exposed to SARS-CoV-2?

Although data are sparse, it appears that being immunosuppressed won't change your threshold for infection. In other words, you would be as susceptible to becoming infected on exposure as someone with a normal immune system.

But counterintuitively, you will be less likely to have a severe disease if you become infected than would a person with a normal immune system. That's because a normal immune system can overreact to the infection. The usual treatment for severe COVID-19 includes immunosuppression to subdue the overreaction. Being already immunosuppressed is in your favor.

What's the difference between autoimmunity and immunosuppression?

Ordinarily, your immune system can tell the difference between your cells and those of an invader. But sometimes a person's immune system begins to make antibodies against that person's own cells or proteins. This can result in a condition called autoimmunity.

Some examples of autoimmune diseases are rheumatoid arthritis, inflammatory bowel disease, lupus, multiple sclerosis, and type 1 diabetes.

These conditions, and many other autoimmune diseases, are treated by medications, such as corticosteroids (often called steroids) to suppress the immune system. In other words, these drugs work by suppressing the immune response that causes the disease—they *cause* immunosuppression.

For example, the immune system sees a transplanted organ as foreign and tries to reject it. So, to prevent rejection, doctors give transplant patients drugs, such as steroids, to suppress the immune system.

With the same medications used to treat both conditions—autoimmune diseases and organ transplantation—it's not surprising that about one person in four who has an immunodeficiency disorder also has an autoimmune disorder, even though the two disorders are different.

COVID-19!

If I get COVID-19 and recover, does that mean I won't get it again?

We don't know the answer to that. We don't have enough data.

But we do know several things.

People who have COVID-19 develop antibodies to the virus, and that suggests—but doesn't prove—immunity might develop.

Some people have recovered from an infection and reportedly have been reinfected—but we don't know if those diagnoses were correct. Nor do we know if the virus stayed around between the two infections; that is, perhaps the person never became virus-free.

Worldwide, a few well-documented repeat infections have been reported. The viruses from the first and second infections were genetically different, so reinfection was confirmed. But those cases may be unusual. The fact that so few reinfections have been documented *suggests* that immunity may follow an infection, and that although reinfection can occur, it doesn't happen often.

Something else we don't know is, if immunity does develop, how long immunity will last. Early studies show declines in antibody levels after recovery.

When we look at the coronaviruses that cause the common cold, immunity lasts only a few months after infection—sometimes perhaps up to a year. Moreover, people can be infected repeatedly with the same coronavirus.

So, bottom line: Only long-term studies will eventually tell us how long immunity will persist after infection with COVID-19. We also don't know at this time how long immunity will last after successful vaccination.

I have a 9-year old son and a 14-year old daughter. Is it true that they're less likely than adults to catch COVID-19?

Yes, children do seem less likely than adults to become infected with SARS-CoV-2, the virus that causes COVID-19.

Research studies suggest why this is.

Receptors are structures on some cells' surface. Virus particles enter cells by attaching to receptors.

As we age, we have more receptors, as shown below (data published by Dr. Bunyavanich and his team). Because children have fewer receptors than adults, the virus has fewer places to attach. That means there are fewer opportunities for the virus to enter children's cells and cause disease.

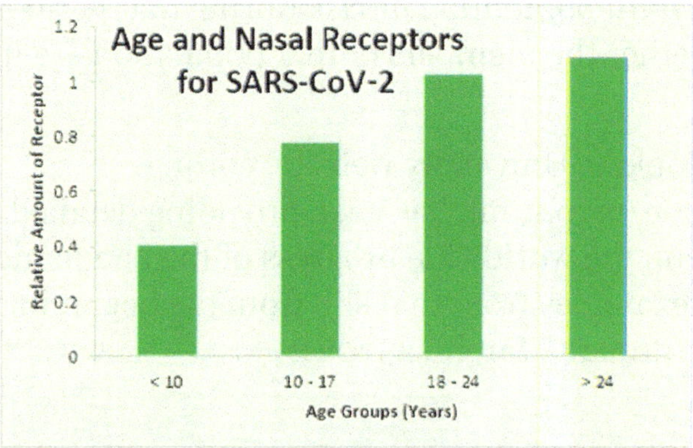

Also, children have lots of colds, some of which are caused by coronaviruses. So children are more likely than adults to develop antibodies to those coronaviruses.

The antibody protection decreases over time. That means that many children are protected from SARS-CoV-2 infection because of the cross-reaction with the common-cold antibodies. This protection could help explain why children are less susceptible to COVID-19, while adults lose the protection they had during childhood.

How do you figure the case fatality rate?

The case fatality (mortality) rate (CFR) is the number of deaths attributed to COVID-19 in a given time period as a fraction of the total cases during that period. The rate is calculated by dividing the number of deaths by the number of confirmed cases in that period.

Number of Deaths ÷ Number of Confirmed Cases = Case Fatality Rate

Similarly, the fatality rate for the population is the number of deaths attributed to COVID-19 in a given time period as a fraction of the *total population at risk* during that period. It doesn't matter whether the members of that population are infected or not.

A Johns Hopkins University website, coronavirus.jhu.edu/map.html, has been providing detailed daily information on the worldwide progress of the pandemic. The table shows examples from that site from the beginning of the pandemic through March 22, 2021:

Location	Confirmed cases	Deaths	Case Mortality Rate (%)
Worldwide	123,308,166	2,716,932	2.2
United States	29,820,276	542,379	1.8
Brazil	11,998,233	294,042	2.5
Mexico	2,195,772	198,036	9.0
India	11,446,081	159,967	1.4
United Kingdom	4,310,195	126,393	2.9
Russia	4,416,226	93,812	2.1

COVID-19!

Basics of Self-Protection

Protecting ourselves from COVID-19
is a ~~serious matter~~—
but sometimes we need to lighten up a bit
and see a little humor in things, as best we can...

MASKS

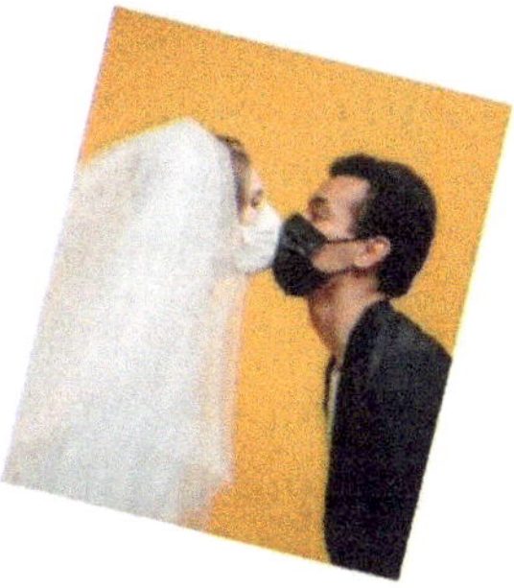

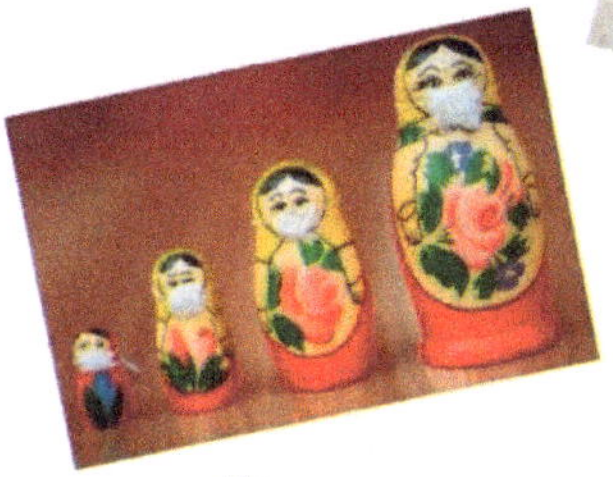

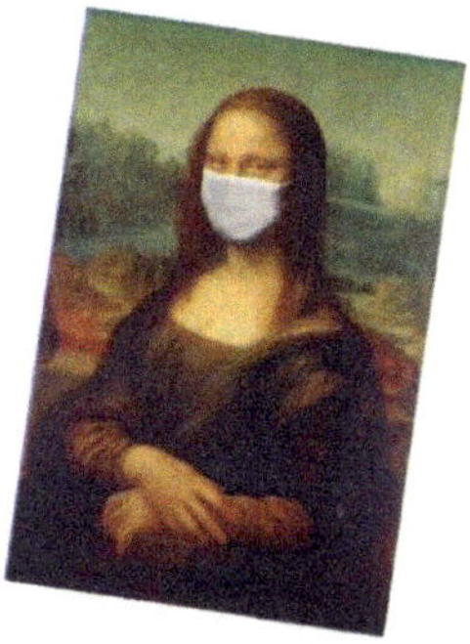

DISTANCE

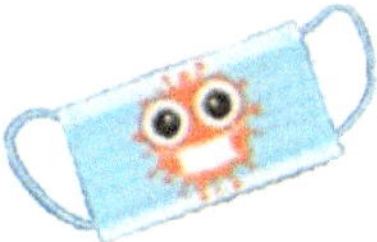

DISINFECTIVES

HANDWASHING

Do I have to wear a mask when I'm just walking down the street?

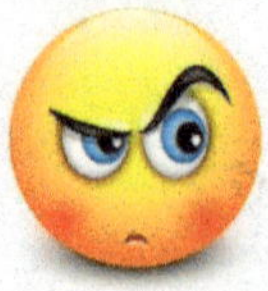

If you're fully vaccinated, you no longer have to wear a mask anywhere, indoors or out. Among the many exceptions are businesses, airlines, or cruise ships that may require you to wear a mask to enter or travel. Local regulations may also require you to continue wearing a mask.

But we also believe in common sense. You have no way of knowing whether people you come in contact with have been vaccinated, and wearing a mask is such a simple and harmless precaution, why not wear one anyhow?

If you would like to cut your risk as much as possible, in addition to your vaccination, wearing a mask when around people you don't know, and who might not be vaccinated, and maintaining at least 6 feet of distance, will help lower your risk level to near zero. But remember, until COVID-19 is no longer around, some risk of getting it remains.

But is it even *safe* to wear a mask? What about interfering with breathing?

I'm glad you asked about safety. Some web posts claim that wearing a mask isn't safe. They're wrong! Lots of advice on the web is bad advice. Ignore it.

As for oxygen problems—stop and think for a minute about what happens during surgery. Teams wear masks throughout surgical procedures—even those lasting many hours. They've been doing that for many decades. Those teams don't lose their ability to concentrate. And they don't become ill or confused from lack of oxygen or an overabundance of carbon dioxide. If they did, just think of the lawsuits!

To obtain evidence, a team from McMaster University in Canada, headed by Dr. Noel Chan, found no difference in oxygen saturation (the amount of oxygen carried by red blood cells) in study volunteers who were wearing masks vs. those who were not.

If I'm fully vaccinated, do I need to maintain my social distance?

As with mask wearing, if you've been fully vaccinated, you can relax some of your social distancing. You can hug your grandchildren again, and shake hands with your friends. If you know they've been vaccinated or have had COVID-19, your risk is very low. But if you don't know their status, you might want to be more cautious.

Even during the first stage of infection, before someone is aware of having been infected, that person may be shedding virus. The virus that causes COVID-19 is spread by aerosols and droplets. These are solid or liquid particles in the air that leave the mouth when we talk. They leave the nose when we breathe out and enter the nose when we breathe in.

We're usually not aware of these tiny particles, not when we produce them and not when someone near us does.

Think of it this way. Imagine everyone is surrounded by a bubble six feet in diameter, open at the bottom.

When we move, so does the bubble. Droplets form when we talk, breathe, cough, or sneeze. The droplets fall to the floor 5 to 10 minutes later, carrying the virus with them.

You don't know who may be shedding virus; to be cautious, stay at least six feet away from everyone. Stay out of everyone's bubble!

Be especially careful if someone is sneezing and isn't wearing a mask. Particles from a sneeze can travel up to 25 feet before settling. A mask cuts that distance down to a few feet.

Mask wearing according to the CDC

Here are some instructions from CDC to help you with your mask.

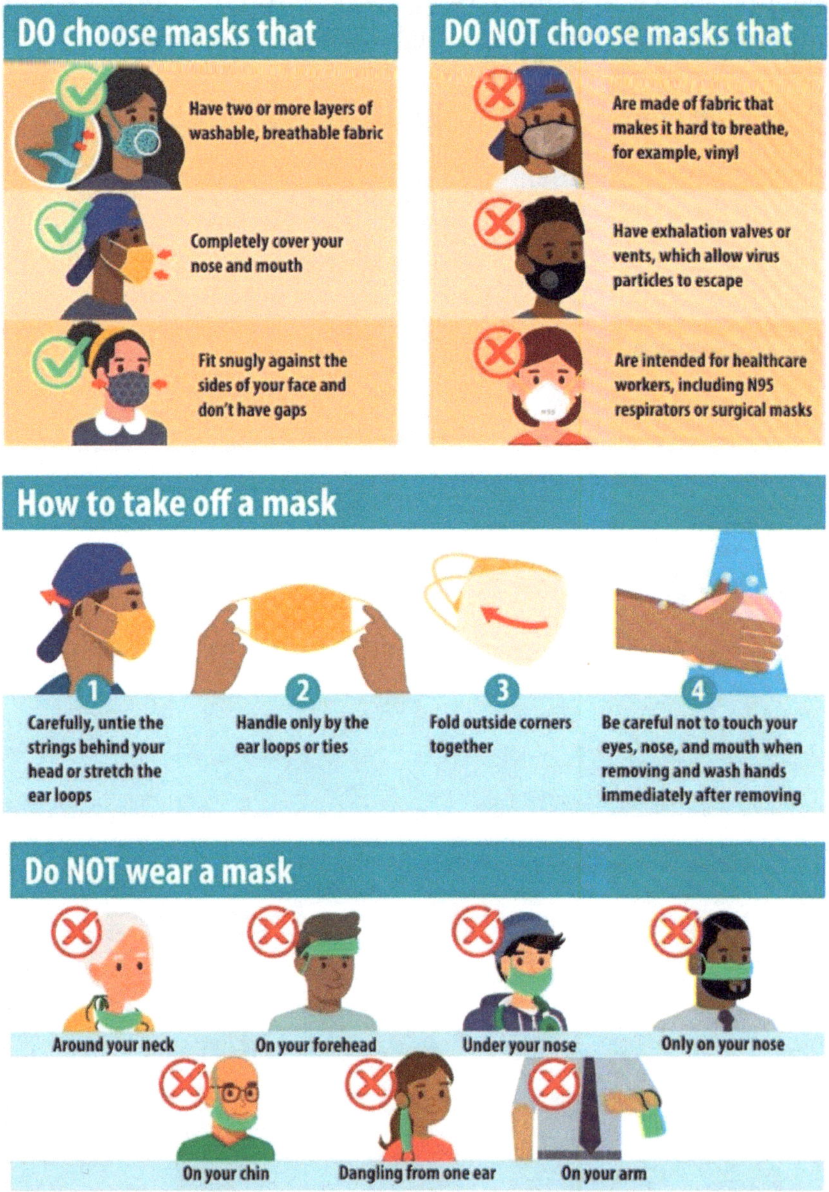

How often do I change masks, and when do I wash them?

The CDC recommends washing masks after each use. If you wash masks in a machine, use detergent and the hottest water temperature possible. If you wash by hand, soak masks in a bleach solution. It's best to dry masks in a hot dryer, because the heat kills most organisms and viruses.

COVID-19!

What do you do when someone who isn't wearing a mask comes near you?

That depends on the circumstances. If it's in a grocery store, what I do is stay away from that person. I maintain at least my six feet of social distance, even though I'm fully vaccinated.

It's best to avoid a confrontational attitude with someone not wearing a mask, especially someone you don't know, because we're not dealing with something logical. Emotional or psychological issues are behind the thinking of many people who refuse to wear a mask. And because the same issues make them not want to be vaccinated, odds are that someone who refuses to wear a mask may also refuse to be vaccinated.

If you want to lower your risk, wear your mask and keep your distance.

What's the difference between droplets and aerosols, and why does it matter?

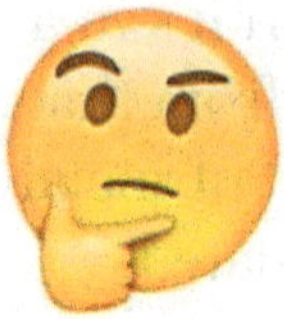

The basic difference between an aerosol and a droplet is the size of the particle. An aerosol is the smaller of the two and floats in the air for a long time before falling or sticking to a surface. A droplet is larger and may fall quickly. Particles in smoke are an example of an aerosol, and a fine mist is an example of droplets.

In dry or warm air, droplets tend to lose their moisture before falling to the ground. They turn into aerosol particles and may remain floating in the air for a long time.

Although general agreement doesn't exist on the difference in size between aerosols and droplets, many people consider aerosol particles to be smaller than 5 micrometers (µm) and droplets to be between 5 and 100 µm. To give some feel for the size of a micrometer (the older term is micron), an average human hair is about 75 µm in diameter. In other words, an aerosol particle is about a fifteenth of the diameter of a human hair.

The difference in size between the two kinds of particles is important for at least two reasons. Aerosols can be carried considerable distances by air currents and have accounted for some widespread outbreaks.

At least two outbreaks have occurred with aerosols that were carried by air currents through sewer pipes into apartments on different floors of apartment buildings. One took place during the SARS outbreak of 2003. Aerosols also accounted for outbreaks during this pandemic: one began in a choir practice and another took place in a restaurant.

How far into the body they go after being inhaled is a second difference between aerosols and droplets. Because they are larger, droplets tend to be trapped in the nose and nasal cavity when someone breathes them in. But aerosols can carry infectious virions—complete virus particles, capable of causing infection—deep into the lungs. Infections in the lungs carry a higher risk of serious or fatal disease than infections in the nose or upper parts of the respiratory tract.

COVID-19!

Why 20 seconds for washing my hands?

You can wash longer if you like, but studies show that washing for 20 seconds is more effective than washing for shorter periods. That's why the CDC recommends a frequent 20-second handwash with soap.

You may find it hard to remember to do this when you get home, so, like me, you might need a reminder—a soap dish placed where you leave your keys, or a note "Wash Hands!" on a table by the door—a way to train yourself to wash your hands *immediately* when you return home. Even from short trips. Even if you just step out to get the mail from the box. Do it before you touch anything in your home. Because every time you're out, you almost certainly touch things someone else has touched.

You're skeptical? Think about the last time you were out. Did you touch a doorknob? An elevator button? The handle to a gas pump? Virus is known to persist a long time on such surfaces.

The problem is that people often touch a contaminated surface and then, soon after, touch their face with their hands or fingers without realizing it.

A study showed that, on average, college students in a classroom touch their face 23 times per hour. Without thinking about it, you can become infected by picking up virus on a surface and transferring it to your nose, mouth, or eyes.

So, why is a 20-second handwashing special?

- Hand washing physically removes most virus particles from the hands
- Soap strips off the fatty envelope that surrounds each virus particle, thus removing the ability of the virus to infect

Should I wear disposable gloves when I go to a store?

Disposable gloves aren't necessary. They aren't even helpful.

Getting virus on your hands won't infect you. You might get infected if you transfer virus from your hands to your face—your eyes, nose, or mouth, as we've talked about—but that can happen whether you're wearing gloves or not.

So, if you choose to wear gloves, wash your hands anyway, *with the gloves on*, before you touch your face. If you can't wash your hands with soap, using sanitizer containing 60% to 85% isopropyl alcohol is second best.

When you remove the gloves, turn them inside out as you pull them off. Put the gloves in the trash, then wash your hands again.

In other words, wearing gloves involves more trouble than it's worth.

What can I do to protect myself when I am in the store?

You can set an alarm on your smart phone before you go into the store to buzz every 10 minutes. That will remind you to wipe your hands with hand sanitizer you carry with you. Do this because you will be touching items and surfaces that others have touched in the store. Then use it on your hands immediately after leaving the store and then again before removing your mask after you're inside your car.

Can I take disinfectants, like bleach or Lysol™, by mouth? Or is it better to inject them?

NEITHER!

NEVER TAKE DISINFECTANTS BY MOUTH, BY GARGLING, OR BY ANY FORM OF INJECTION!

Disinfectants, such as bleach or Lysol, are effective for eliminating infectious virus from many surfaces. They get rid of virions from many surfaces we routinely touch; doorknobs, handrails, handles of supermarket carts, to mention a few.

But disinfectants are dangerous, even fatal, if taken internally. By "taken internally," we mean allowed entry to the body—***by mouth, or by injection, or by any other means.*** Even if allowed inside the body, disinfectants would be totally ineffective against the virus.

Hand sanitizer, if taken internally, is extremely toxic. Like disinfectants, *hand sanitizer is not for internal use.* Ingredients in hand sanitizer will damage the throat, stomach, and intestine.

We're aware of a case that makes the point. A woman became ill after swallowing two teaspoons of hand sanitizer every day, mistakenly thinking it would prevent COVID-19. Excellent hospital care saved her life, but her digestive tract was severely damaged. Other reports describe deaths of people who have swallowed disinfectants.

School Reopening

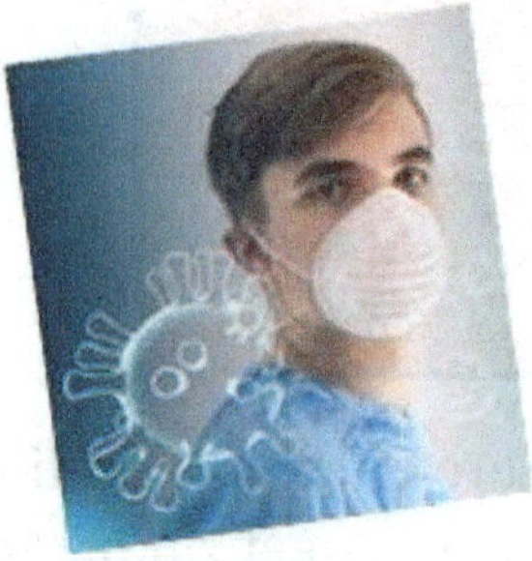

Schools Reopen:
COVID-19 Cases Crop Up

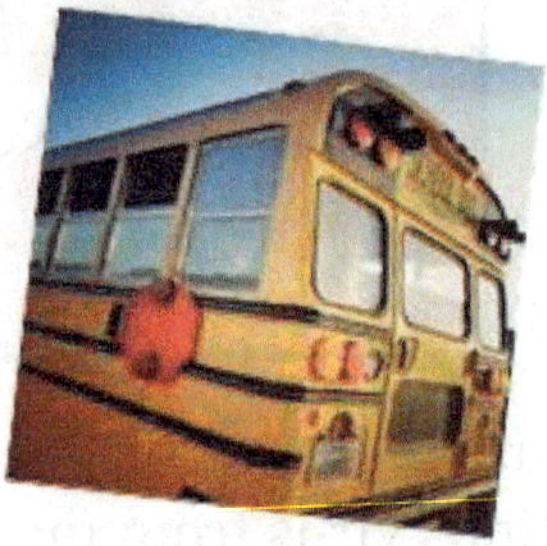

U.S. breaks August record for new coronavirus cases

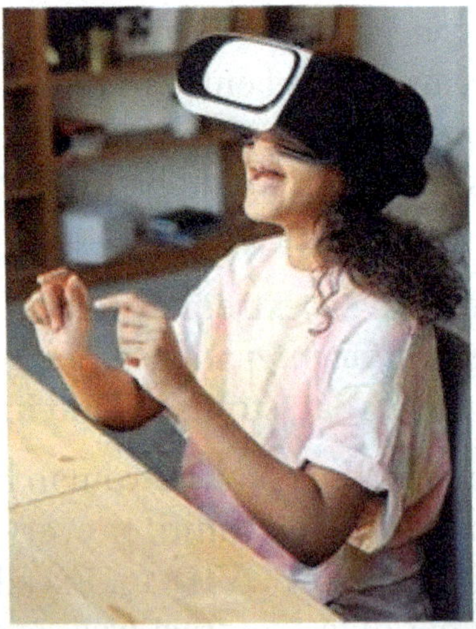

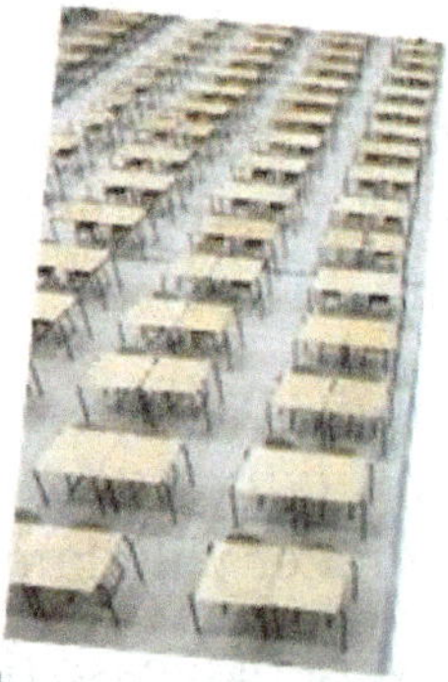

Where are the kids?

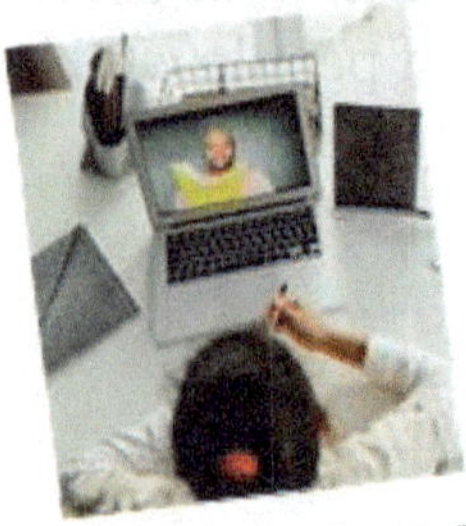

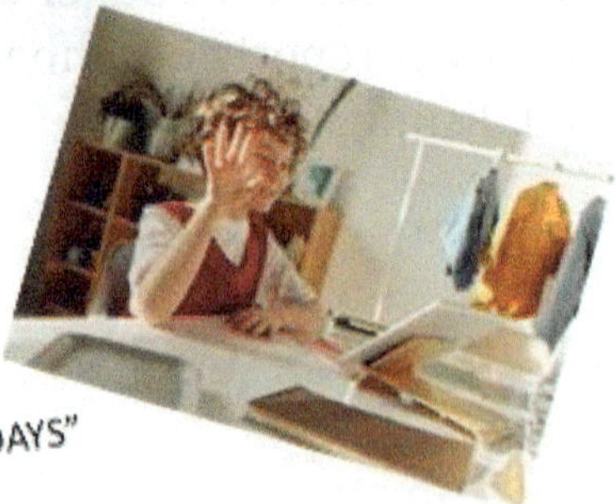

"SCHOOL DAYS, SCHOOL DAYS"

How will our state decide about letting kids return to school?

Anthony Fauci, MD, director of the National Institute of Allergy and Infectious Diseases, shared his thoughts about school openings in a televised August 13, 2020 interview with Rhode Island Governor Gina Raimondo, carried on Facebook Live.

In his usual practical approach, Dr. Fauci commented on public health officials' designated zones—red, yellow, or green—as key factors in school return. Green zones have a test-positivity rate of less than 5% and fewer than 10 cases per 100,000 residents, he noted; with contact tracing and other factors in place, schools in green zones probably should be allowed to open.

Yellow zones have a 5% to 10% test-positivity rate and 10 to 100 cases per 100,000. Red zones have a test-positivity rate above 10% and more than 100 cases per 100,000 residents. "The best way for a state, city, or county that's red to get their children back to school is to do what's needed to become yellow, and yellow to do what's needed to become green," Dr. Fauci commented.

He advised red states wanting to reopen schools that they have a choice—"either close the bars or close the schools," he said—tossing out a line that has since been widely quoted. He equated a state where people were getting together in bars with a state that would probably remain red. In contrast, a state that was doing something to improve things likely was one that could transition to yellow, or even green.

He cautioned that no matter what, some cases of COVID-19 will continue to appear, even in the green areas, because "nothing is 100 percent."

Because of the success of the vaccines, all schools in the U.S. are expected to open for in-person learning in the fall of 2021.

COVID-19!

Our school is giving us a choice: in-person or remote classes. How should we decide?

My wife and I haven't had to think about that personally, because our children have been out of school for a long time. So, for some guidance, I checked to see what a fellow MD had posted on the subject. He's Sanjay Gupta, MD, CNN Chief Medical Correspondent, and the father of three girls of school age.

Dr. Gupta mentioned that more than half of the largest school districts in the country had decided on virtual learning, but the school in his district left the choice up to the family. His daughters wanted very much to attend in person, so he had to do some research.

He began by visiting the head of the girls' school and asking what precautions the school would be taking. The school checked out well; it was following CDC recommendations—mask mandate, physical distancing, stations for hand-hygiene, frequent surface-disinfecting, lunches in the classroom, and plans for outdoor classes when weather permits. No mass gatherings. COVID-19 tests for all students, faculty, and staff before school opening.

Next, the family reviewed the data on COVID-19 transmission by children and looked at the rate of new cases in their area.

That's when the first problem appeared. Local requirements for returning to school called for fewer than 100 new cases per 100,000 people during the previous 14 days. The actual rate in their area was much higher—316 cases. Not a good number.

Nor did the county data meet the criteria from the Coronavirus Task Force—two periods of a downtrend in documented cases, with no patients requiring crisis care.

Finally, Dr. Gupta noted that the state's rate of positive test results during the seven days ending August 10 was 11.3%, based on data from the COVID-19 Tracking Project—indicating insufficient testing.

The family's decision: even though the school was open, the girls wouldn't be returning on an in-person basis, at least not right away.

https://www.wral.com/coronavirus/dr-sanjay-gupta-why-i-am-not-sending-my-kids-back-to-school/19231701/

The data Dr. Gupta unearthed left the family with little choice.

When your family is making the decision about school attendance, here are factors to consider:

How well is your school minimizing the crowding and mixing of students? How well is it enforcing the basics of mask-wearing, social distancing, and personal hygiene? What about hand-washing?

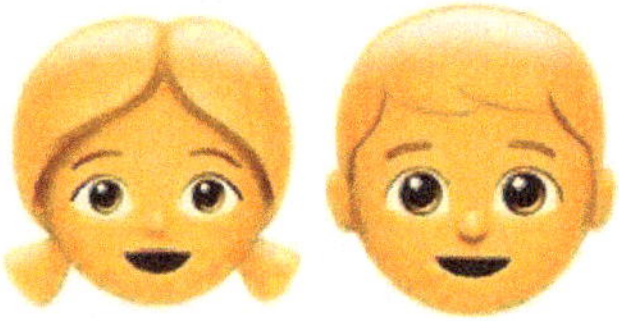

Are classrooms well ventilated? Are windows kept open when weather permits? Are desks well separated? Are kids, teachers, and staff required to wear masks—and, if so, is the regulation enforced? Are there plenty of hand-hygiene stations? Are surfaces disinfected frequently? Is the school among those that have installed a plexiglass shield around each student's desk area?

Does the school stagger starting times, recess times, and lunch breaks to help separate children of different grades?

Personal factors are every bit as important as precautions the school is taking. What is your home and neighborhood situation? Do you live close enough to the school for the child to walk safely both ways, or will someone drive—or walk with—the child? If not, how crowded are the school buses? Do buses have an adult present to monitor the kids, or is the driver responsible for maintaining discipline—and enforcing mask-wearing?

Is there anyone at home who is especially susceptible to COVID-19 and thus could be at risk if the child becomes infected, even if the child is asymptomatic? "Others" include siblings, parents, elderly grandparents, or anyone who has a chronic condition or is at special risk.

If you've considered all the factors we've discussed, but neither decision—onsite or remote learning—seems a clear choice, reading Dr. Anthony Fauci's comments in the question directly below may be helpful. If you live in a state or community with a high prevalence of COVID-19 cases, you may decide that remote learning is the better choice, even if your school is open. If you live in a community with low prevalence of COVID-19 and few hospitalizations, you may decide to let your child attend in-person learning.

Everyone knows how important in-person schooling is for our children's social and mental development. Opening schools as early as possible is a worthy goal, but when you're responsible for young lives, you need to make sure that when children return, they do so safely. Schooling needs to be not just a rewarding experience but a safe one as well; safe for students, safe for teachers and school personnel, and safe for the adults who are important in students' lives.

Our high school is switching to something called *K-12online*. What's that all about?

An article in *JAMA Pediatrics* discusses K-12online in detail.

https://COVID-1919.elsevierpure.com/en/publications/k-12-virtual-schooling-COVID-19-and-student-success

We weren't familiar with K-12online, but now that COVID-19 has elevated remote learning to a key concept, we've done a little research. We'll pass along some of what we learned from the *JAMA Pediatrics* article, cited above, and from other sources.

K-12online programs offer general education and special education curricula for students from kindergarten through 12th grade. Curricula are designed specifically for online use, and many teachers have been specially trained in the K-12online program.

When elementary school students enroll in a K-12online program, parents usually need to be involved in the students' work. But students at middle schools and high schools often work independently, taking part in group and individualized learning programs by email, telephone, or video. Usually, it's not necessary for students and teachers to be online at the same time, so students have flexibility as to when and where they take part in the online programs.

That said, parents do need to do their own homework. Some K-12 online schools are much better than others; it's important for parents to check reviews of the local school, along with data about the school's educational outcomes. This information may be available in local newspapers or you may need to talk with the school's superintendent or principal.

The *JAMA Pediatrics* article points out that students in these programs "need to be motivated, organized, and supported," and that success, in part, depends on students' access to instructional support and to the internet.

COVID-19!

An advantage of virtual K-12 schooling lies in helping children with special health care needs—for example, by providing the practical flexibility some students require, especially those who often miss onsite classes because of illness or health care visits.

How can I tell how well my child would do with online learning?

The article in *JAMA Pediatrics,* mentioned above, offers questions for parents to think about regarding online learning. Answering those questions may help you decide whether your child is ready for online learning. They'll also help you assess the online school.

The first four questions concern the child's readiness; the questions that follow focus on the virtual school.

Can your child

- independently adhere to a study schedule and finish assignments on time?
- ask for help and communicate effectively with a teacher by telephone, text, email, or video?

Does your child

- have an innate drive to learn skills, gather knowledge, and finish assignments?
- have basic skills in math, reading, writing, and computer literacy?

≈ How will the virtual school share student information with the local school district?

≈ Is the virtual school accredited?

≈ Does it comply with state licensure requirements and other standards for K-12 educators?

≈ What does the school expect from parents and caregivers?

≈ What support does it offer children with special needs?

≈ Do instructional materials reflect Universal Design for Learning (UDL) standards?

≈ What tech equipment do students need for the program? Who will provide it?

(The UDL website defines UDL Guidelines as a tool used in the implementation of Universal Design for Learning, a framework to improve and optimize teaching and learning for all people, based on scientific insights into how humans learn.)

If my 5th grader goes back to school, will he catch the virus and transmit it to someone in the family?

Of course, children can and do develop COVID-19, although studies so far suggest that they're less likely to do so than adults. It seems that children usually have only minor symptoms but can transmit the virus to others at about the same rate as adults. And kids pass the virus not just to their young friends, but to adults as well. So if you have older adults (such as the kids' grandparents) at home where your kids could expose them, you might want to consider whether you want to take that risk.

Schools that have opened for in-person attendance have reported mixed results in terms of COVID-19 outbreaks. Some schools continue to be open, but others have closed again.

Coping With Isolation

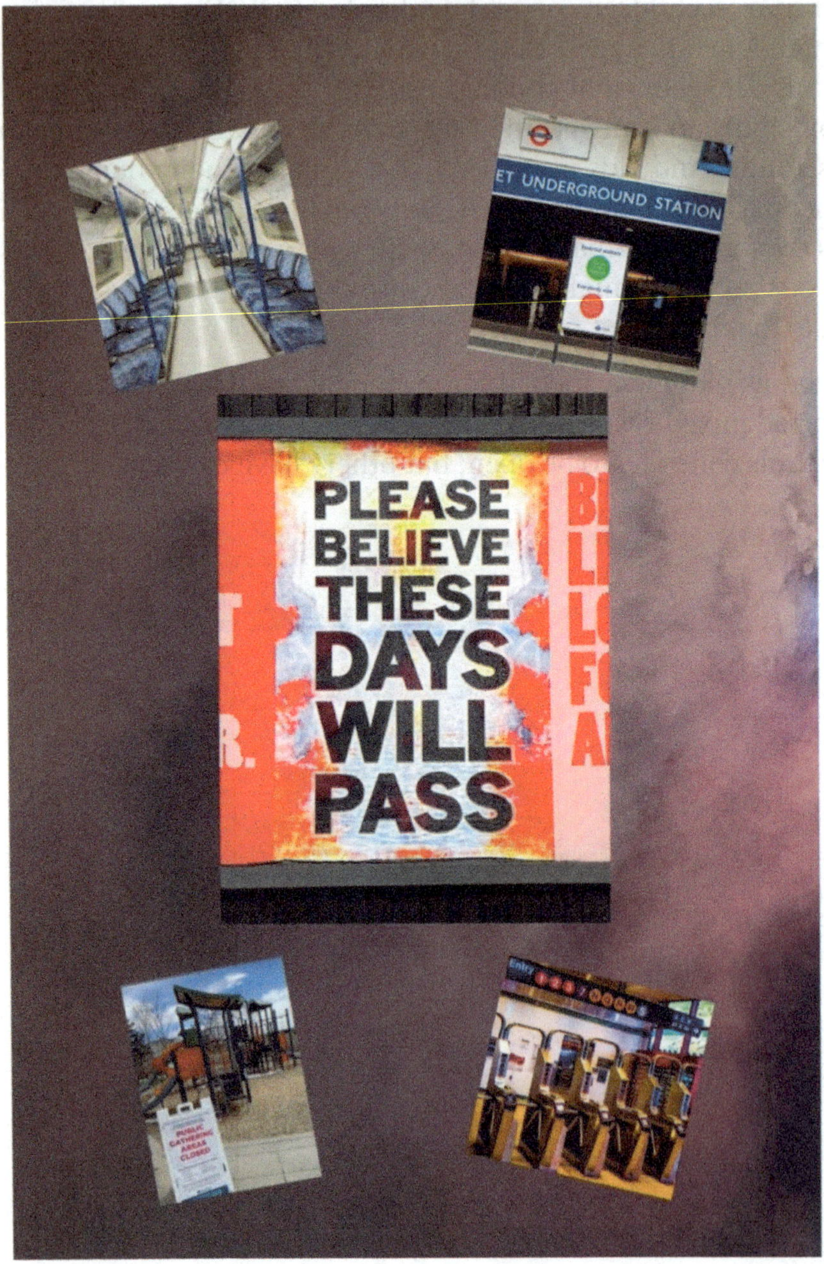

I have a mild case of COVID-19 and need to isolate at home. How can I keep my family safe?

Unfortunately, the only sure way to protect your family is to isolate yourself. That means confining yourself to a bedroom and bathroom reserved for your use only. Air from your rooms should not be allowed to enter the rest of the house.

Family can leave prepared meals at your door, with a pleasant heads-up: a welcome knock. A special treat or a note on the tray can help lighten your day.

Obvious things to help you pass the time—a TV, laptop computer, and books—don't substitute for contact with your loved ones, but frequent phone conversations will help. If you're set up for Zoom or a similar service, seeing and talking with your loved ones can be a real morale booster.

You'll need to confine yourself for at least 10 days after your symptoms started, after you've had no fever for at least 24 hours without the help of fever-reducing medications, and when your other symptoms are improving. When your isolation time ends, be sure to check with your doctor to find out whether you should have a COVID-19 test.

I've just been told that someone I've been in close contact with has been diagnosed with COVID-19, and I'm not fully vaccinated. What should I do?

You need to call your doctor's office or your local health department for instructions. *But before you call*, make sure that you *did have close contact* as authorities redefined it on October 21, 2020: You were within six feet of an infected person for a cumulative total of at least 15 minutes during a 24-hour period.

Experts defined the 24-hour period (total of 24 hours) as beginning two days before the infected contact's onset of illness (or, for asymptomatic patients, two days before collection of the test specimen) and ending the first day of isolation.

Note that examples of a 15-minute exposure could be three 5-minute exposures, five 3-minute exposures, and so forth.

- For 15 minutes or more, you were within 6 feet of someone who has COVID-19, or
- You provided care at home to someone with COVID-19, or
- You had direct physical contact with the person (you hugged or kissed), or
- You shared eating or drinking utensils, or
- The person sneezed, coughed, or in some way transferred respiratory droplets to you

As for what you should do, here's what the CDC recommends:

- Stay home for 10 days after your last contact with a person who has COVID-19, and
- Watch for fever (100.4 F or higher), cough, shortness of breath, or other symptoms of COVID-19, and
- If possible, stay away from others, especially people at high risk for becoming severely ill with COVID-19

COVID-19!

For a list of conditions associated with higher risk, go to https://www.cdc.gov/coronavirus/2019-ncov/need-extra-precautions/index.html?CDC_AA_refVal=https%3A%2F%2Fwww.cdc.gov%2Fcoronavirus%2F2019-ncov%2Fneed-extra-precautions%2Fpeople-at-increased-risk.html

COVID-19!

I was in close contact last week with someone who has now come down with COVID-19, but two months ago I was diagnosed with the disease myself. Do I need to quarantine? Or get tested again?

No. People who have tested positive for COVID-19 do not need to quarantine—or get tested again—during the three months after they receive positive test results.

For people who have recovered from a SARS-CoV-2 infection, a positive PCR test result during the 90 days after the illness began probably doesn't indicate a reinfection. So, if someone remains *asymptomatic* during those 90 days, retesting probably won't provide any useful information. That is true even if that person had close contact with an infected person.

But, if symptoms develop during the 90 days, and no other condition—such as influenza—seems to account for the symptoms, a caregiver may decide, perhaps in consultation with a health care provider, to evaluate the person for SARS-CoV-2 reinfection. Isolation may be warranted during the evaluation, especially if the symptoms developed after close contact with an infected person.

I'm in isolation. I developed symptoms after I tested positive. Do I need to be tested so I can leave isolation?

In general, you can leave isolation under the following conditions:

- At least 10 days have passed since the appearance of your first symptoms; **and**
- You haven't had a fever for at least 24 hours and have not taken any fever-reducing medication; **and**
- There's an improvement in symptoms of COVID-19, other than with your senses of taste and smell

(Isolation can end even if you haven't regained your senses of taste and smell, because these senses sometimes fail to return until weeks or months after recovery. Fatigue also can persist.)

As for testing, the CDC no longer recommends a test-based strategy for deciding when to discontinue isolation, except in certain circumstances. The reason: newly available data indicate that people who have had—and recovered from—COVID-19 may have low levels of viral RNA in their bodies for as long as three months after diagnosis. If these people are retested during those first three months, the test result may be positive—*even though those people aren't infectious and cannot spread COVID-19.*

I tested positive for COVID-19, but I haven't had any symptoms. When can I leave isolation?

If you continue to be without symptoms, you can be with other people:

- 10 days after the date of your positive test

Your caregiver may recommend repeat testing for COVID-19, so you could try to leave isolation a bit earlier. If so, as mentioned above, you can be around others after you receive two negative test results in a row, from tests done at least 24 hours apart. Of course, you should continue to wear a mask when in public, maintain social distance, and wash your hands frequently.

I was severely ill with COVID-19. How long must I stay in isolation?

If you were admitted to a hospital and needed oxygen, your health care provider may recommend that you stay in isolation longer than 10 days—possibly as long as 20 days—after your first symptoms appeared, and you may need to finish your period of isolation at home.

Your healthcare provider may recommend that you undergo repeat testing for COVID-19. If so, you can be around others after you receive two negative tests results in a row, from tests done at least 24 hours apart. That could give you a chance to end your isolation earlier than you could under the criteria listed above, depending on how much time is needed for test scheduling and report delivery.

I started quarantine because of contact with my partner, who has COVID-19. But one day he needed help, so we had close contact again. What should I do now?

You need to restart your quarantine, beginning with the day of your new close contact. The same would be true if anyone else in your household comes down with COVID-19.

My partner is extremely ill with COVID-19, and I need to give him constant care.

You need to avoid contact with other people until 14 days after your partner has met the criteria for ending isolation. This advice applies also to people who lack a separate room for isolation and to people who live in extremely close quarters and cannot maintain a physical distance of 6 feet.

I tested positive for COVID-19, and I have a weakened immune system. When can I leave isolation?

If your immune system is weakened—that is, if you're immunocompromised—because of a health condition or medication you're taking—you might need to stay in isolation longer than 10 days. Ask your health care provider for guidance.

COVID-19!

If I'm going to get COVID-19 anyway, why not go out NOW with friends, eat at restaurants, have fun? If I get infected, I'll just get it over with!

Instead, how about waiting? Waiting will give you two possibilities, and that's better than playing today's odds. One possibility: someone comes up with a treatment that works; then, if you get COVID-19, you won't be as sick, and you'll be sick for a shorter time. The second possibility: if you're able to be vaccinated, you will be safe from COVID-19 altogether.

COVID-19!

I'm getting tired of staying home, avoiding everything. Can I go out for some fun?

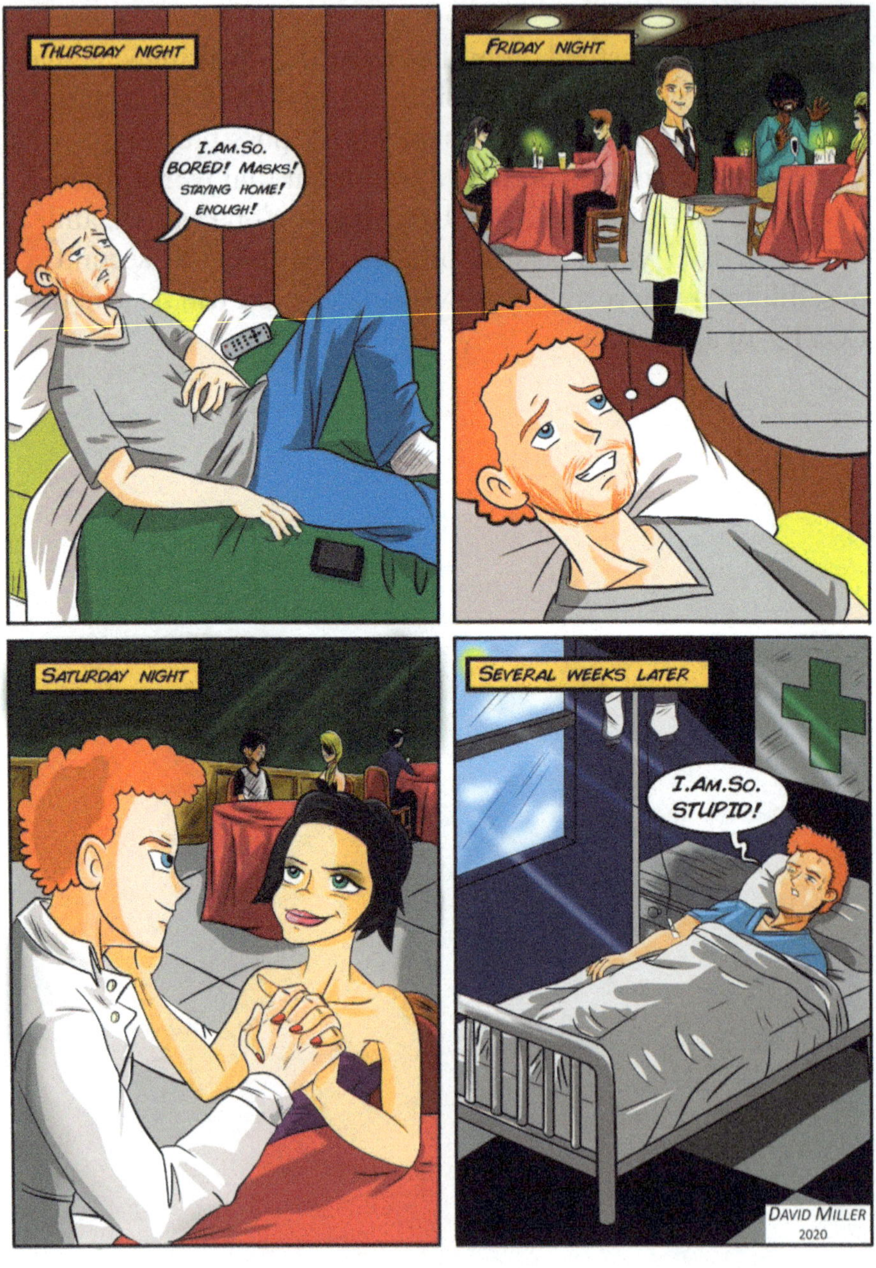

Maybe I'm starting to get depressed.

I get it; I hear you. And I can help. This is no time to give up doing the things that help keep you safe, but I don't see any reason you couldn't loosen up a little. And here's why and how.

There are some tools out there to help you, like a chart that ranks ordinary activities by risk level (https://www.texmed.org/TexasMedicineDetail.aspx?id=53977). The chart comes from the Texas Medical Association (TMA), a group of 53,000 physicians and medical students in Texas. It's put together by doctors from the across the state. So, although this chart isn't perfect, it's got some power behind it.

A representative from the TMA explained to *Newsweek* that the numbers don't represent percentages. The ranking is based on how hard it is to maintain social distancing and other preventive steps in the situations listed. For example, it's easy to wear a mask and maintain distance when pumping gas—ranked 2—but not so easy to do that at a food buffet, ranked 8.

Take a look. Stay in the Low Risk or Moderate-Low Risk areas, where you have plenty of choices. You could pick up a meal from your favorite restaurant. Go to a library or museum. Even play golf! Take a walk with someone—even in a busy downtown area, or by the beach. (Just don't forget your mask; keep your social distance, and wash your hands often and thoroughly.)

But—don't even *think* about getting your hair cut at a barber shop or salon or going to an amusement park. The chart ranks those as high-risk activities. But also keep in mind that these and other activities vary in their risk depending on precautions taken, because some risks can be reduced to acceptable levels.

I need to know when I can go back to work—but I want to go back safely.

The decision to permit businesses to reopen will be up to federal, state, and local governments. Depending on the nature of the business, however, some businesses will choose to remain closed, or to continue to have their employees work from home. Those that choose to reopen can implement the lessons learned since the pandemic started.

But you don't need to go along with the decision. You should not go out or to work until you personally feel safe. That's true even if the government has relaxed or lifted stay-at-home orders and other restrictions. You need to base your decision on your age, your medical conditions and overall health, the age and health of others in your household, and your location—that is, whether you are in a viral "hotspot."

Remember: If you believe restrictions have been lifted too soon in your area and you don't feel safe, *you need to wait.*

Unfortunately, the nature of your job may require onsite work—or you'll lose your job. In that case, you need to adhere to all the safety precautions to minimize your risk at your job.

Here's a summary of the current federal guidelines for reopening.

Based on local disease conditions:

- A two-week period of fewer reports of influenza-like illnesses, ***and***
- A two-week period of decreased reporting of COVID-19-like cases

Based on confirmed cases:

- A two-week period of decreasing positive cases, ***or***

- A two-week period of decreasing positive tests as a percentage of total tests (to make sure that the number of positive tests isn't rising simply because more testing is going on)

Based on robustness of health care facilities:

- Hospitals in the area must be able to safely treat all patients who need hospitalization without resorting to crisis standards of care
- Facilities must have the capability in place to test all health care workers for virus and antibody

After the above gating criteria are met, governors and local officials can proceed to reopening in phases as laid out in the guidelines.

I'm tired of cooking. Can I safely eat packaged foods?

The food inside the package should be safe to eat. It's extremely unlikely that any virus particles would be inside. Even if virus particles are inside, cooking the food will inactivate the virus, whether the food was stored in the refrigerator or freezer.

The outside of the package is a different story. Virus can stay infective on a package's surface for at least nine days at room temperature, as long as a month in the refrigerator, and indefinitely in the freezer.

So you should disinfect the outside of the package if you want to be especially cautious, as you might be if you have conditions that increase your risk, or if others in your household are in a high-risk category. On the side of saying that less caution is okay, few if any infections have been caused by contaminated food or its packaging.

Can I safely eat carryout food from a restaurant? What if I cook the food?

According to the CDC, the COVID-19 virus is carried in respiratory droplets from an infected person to another person, who then becomes infected. CDC adds, "Currently there is no evidence to support transmission of COVID-19 associated with food."

To dig a little deeper, saying there is no evidence doesn't mean that transmission through food can't happen—just that nobody has tested to find out. So let's look at a few possibilities.

A carryout usually comes in a paper or plastic bag, packaged by a restaurant cook. The food typically is hot. The food itself is probably perfectly safe to eat, assuming it is hot, unlike a take-out salad. Heat quickly inactivates viruses, and SARS-CoV-2 is no exception.

But what if the cook or others at the restaurant had virus on their hands and spread the virus to the package? Yes, you could pick up virus, get the virus on your hands, and touch your face, resulting in an infection.

But there's a very small chance of that. To reduce the odds even more, consider the package contaminated.

As soon as restaurants reopen, I want to go out and celebrate!

I can't tell you if it's safe to do that, because there's no clear answer. Many factors are involved, including whether you're fully vaccinated.

For instance, would you be inside the restaurant or outside? If inside, what is the air circulation pattern? Can you be in a place directly in front of an air supply vent, so that the air that circulates to you hasn't passed by any other diners? Does the table layout provide for distance between diners?

We've learned a lot from what happened after a lunch party at a restaurant in China. The party took place on January 24, 2020, early in the pandemic. That was before much was known about the pandemic and how important it is to maintain distance.

Family A in the figure below had just arrived from Wuhan. Patient A1 developed symptoms later that day and was hospitalized. Other diners developed the disease on the dates shown. The virus spread easily from A1 to the others because of the air circulation from the air conditioner. Note that other diners in the restaurant and staff members did not become infected; they were outside the path of the recirculating air.

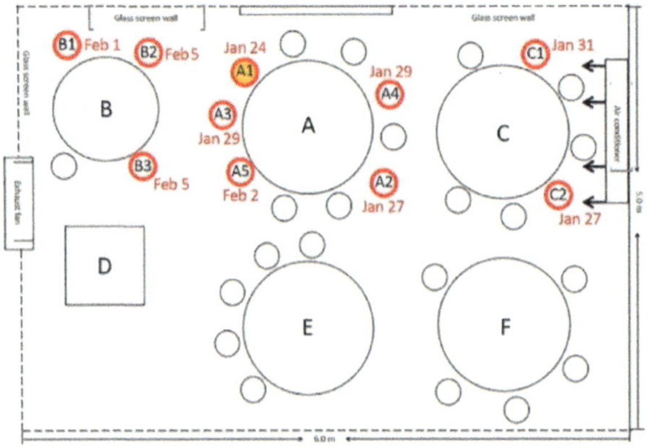

COVID-19!

Based on studies we've seen, we did not dine inside restaurants until we were fully vaccinated, although we ordered takeout meals.

We're not encouraging anyone to dine indoors unless they are fully vaccinated. You should also check out the restaurant air circulation and table arrangement. The story above says why.

COVID-19!

Travel

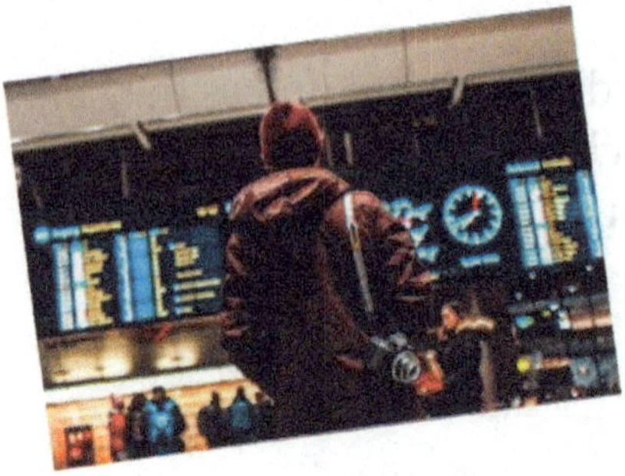

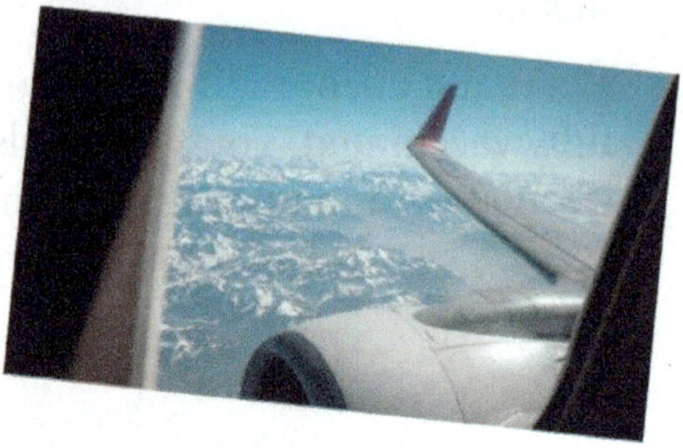

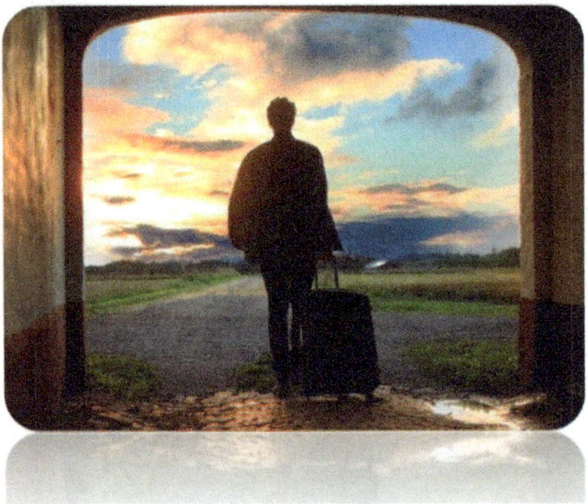

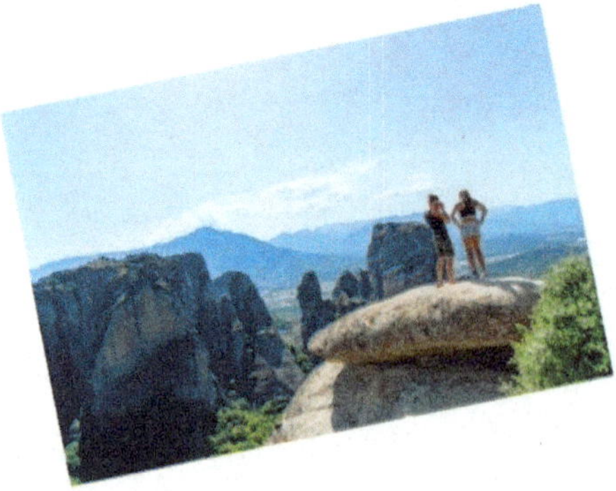

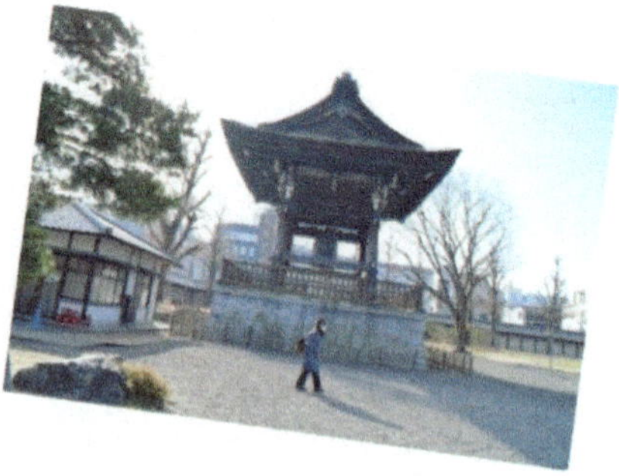

COVID-19!

What precautions should I take for my upcoming flight?

Don't fly unless you absolutely must. If you must fly, take every possible precaution, including being vaccinated.

When choosing your airline, check COVID-19 policies. Some airlines have made flights reasonably safe; they're keeping some seats vacant to create social distancing; and they're requiring everyone to wear a mask and have a temperature check before boarding.

Of course, airlines say it's safe to fly. Although ventilation systems have been improved over the years and many modern aircraft have high efficiency particulate air (HEPA) filters for the recirculated air, the filters are often poorly maintained, and unfiltered air can bypass the filter. And remember that you'll be on the flight for at least an hour and many times that for an overseas flight, so your risk of exposure can be very high.

While the plane is loading, strangers will be close to you in the aisle, often talking loudly. During your flight, remain seated as much as possible with your mask on. If there is an air outlet overhead, direct the nozzle at your head with maximum air flow. This will help form a protective shield around you that will help keep droplets and aerosols from other passengers from getting into your space, but it won't protect you from contaminated, recirculated air. Unfortunately, many passengers remove their masks after the plane is in the air. Don't forget, you'll be sitting close to strangers, even if you're surrounded by empty seats.

Getting to and from the plane is possibly the riskiest part of a trip. Carefully time your arrival at the airport and at the gate to minimize waiting time.

Avoid shuttle buses if at all possible because they tend to be crowded and often have poor ventilation.

COVID-19!

Keeping adequate distance from others is difficult in an airport, but do your best. Wear a mask, of course, and when walking through lobbies and concourses and sitting in waiting rooms, stay away from anyone who isn't masked.

Carry a bottle of hand sanitizer and use it frequently. Sanitizing wipes are useful but are sometimes in short supply; you can make your own by putting paper towels in a small plastic bag with a zipper closure and wetting the towels with rubbing (isopropyl) alcohol (60% to 85% percent). It's a good idea to carry the bag with you and use the towels to wipe the armrests in your seat and any other surfaces you will touch.

If I drive instead of fly, what precautions should I take?

If you're fully vaccinated, driving can be safer than flying, at least with respect to SARS-CoV-2 infections.

If your trip requires an overnight stay, can you put up with sleeping in your car in a relatively busy, brightly lit rest area, instead of staying in a motel? It may not be comfortable, but it's safer, at least from a COVID-19 standpoint.

(You'll see tips about how to improve the safety of a motel room in the next section.)

You can get your meals at drive-through restaurants.

When you stop for gasoline, be sure to wipe the fueling nozzle with disinfectant before using it, and wash your hands or use hand sanitizer after fueling.

Public restrooms are a problem. We believe that they're quite risky, but a preliminary internet search didn't reveal much support for our view. It was only when we accessed the primary literature—scientific papers written by PhD and MD researchers—that we found data that back our concerns and substantiate concerns about health risks.

The problems involve aerosols and droplets that are released and take to the air when a toilet is flushed—not just the toilet you flushed, but toilets flushed several hours before you even entered the washroom.

We'll be looking into this and writing more about it, but in the meantime we have several suggestions. Take alcohol wipes into the washroom, and use them on the door to the stall and on the flush knob on the toilet. Also use a wipe or toilet paper to touch the water faucet handles. Never turn off the handles with your bare hands. Spend as little time in the washroom as possible. Wash your hands before you leave.

COVID-19!

What if there's an electric hand dryer but no paper towels? Here is an area where you'll find *lots* of opinions if you do an internet search. The problem is that the opinions don't agree. To try to shed some light on this issue, Dr. Kelly Reynolds and others at the University of Arizona surveyed many publications containing research results comparing the two ways for drying hands in public restrooms and found no consistent differences in the two methods.

Our advice, don't dry your hands with either method. Instead, use an alcohol wipe or let your hands dry outside the restroom.

When you leave the washroom, use another alcohol wipe to open the door. And, when you're back in the car, apply hand sanitizer.

A final suggestion: consider purchasing a urinary device and avoiding public washrooms. Amazon lists many types of devices, some costing less than $20. Even some models for very young kids are listed.

And always remember the four basics: Be vaccinated, wear your mask when out of the car, wash your hands for 20 seconds, and keep as much distance from others as you can, but at least six feet.

What about staying in a hotel or motel? Could someone have left the virus on light switches, bathroom faucet handles, doorknobs, TV remotes, and other places?

Yes, that's quite likely—*if* someone infected with the virus stayed in the room during the two weeks or so before you arrived.

The virus that causes COVID-19 can remain infective on various surfaces for up to four weeks at room temperature. The number of infective virus particles continually decreases during that time. That's what we know. What we don't know is what this means in terms of your risks of coming down with COVID-19 if you stay in the room. We just don't have the data yet.

So here's what I suggest. As soon as you enter a motel room, wipe surfaces with 60 to 80 percent alcohol. Or, you can use bleach, diluted to between 1:10 to 1:50; that translates to 1 tablespoon of standard bleach in 5 to 25 ounces of water. If you have neither alcohol nor bleach, wash faucet handles and other surfaces with soap and water.

COVID-19!

Should I take a cruise now? Prices are probably down.

U.S. cruise companies closed their operations and plans for resuming sailings vary widely from company to company. Precautions planned by the various cruise lines also vary, regarding preboarding testing of passengers, for example, and requiring proof of vaccination. And remember, even if the test results for all passengers immediately before boarding reveal no infections, a passenger who had been infected up to two days before would have a negative test result and could board and infect others during the cruise.

My advice is that cruising remains unsafe. If only one person on board is an asymptomatic carrier—that is, infected but without showing symptoms—the virus could quickly take hold and spread throughout the tight quarters of a cruise ship.

When that happens, people are confined to cabins, although it's not clear how the ship will deal with passengers who are fully vaccinated. Imagine being quarantined in a tiny room—a Google search revealed that a roomy standard cabin is about 170 to 190 square feet, but some cabins are only 85 to 100 square feet. For comparison, the average hotel room is 330 square feet.

Cruises also differ in their planned ports-of-call. Some ports are closed to visitors, and some do not allow Americans to disembark because of the high positivity rate in the U.S. Canada has banned cruises until March 2022.

https://www.frommers.com/tips/cruise/cabin-clues-how-to-choose-the-right-room-at-sea

https://www.usatoday.com/story/travel/roadwarriorvoices/2015/11/04/hotel-rooms-20-years-ago-were-twice-as-large-as-some-of-todays-offerings/83847338/

So how big a risk do we have of catching the virus on a cruise ship?

As of mid-May, 2020, at least 40 cruise ships out of about 315 worldwide reported at least one case of COVID-19 on board during a cruise. The six ships with the highest number of cases are shown in the table, adapted from the table of 40 ships in Wikipedia. The Wikipedia article also noted that not all ships or operating companies have been entirely transparent or honest in their reporting, so we're not relying on their reports.

Ship	Passengers + Crew	Tests	Cases	Dead
Ruby Princess			≥852	21
Diamond Princess	3711	3618	712	14
Celebrity Apex	1407	1444	224	
Costa Atlantica	623	~50%	148	
Greg Mortimer	217	all	128	1
Grand Princess	3533	1103	122	7

Because of this history of cases and the mortality data, it's best to delay taking a cruise until at least two weeks after your chosen cruise ship has been free of COVID-19 cases. The report of no cases should come from sources other than the cruise lines. But remember that asymptomatic infected passengers can test negative at boarding time, yet transmit the virus after a few days into the cruise.

When you consider the high number of passengers on a cruise ship, which increases the chance that one of them may be an asymptomatic carrier, and the close quarters that make social distancing very difficult, I believe the risk is very high. Even if you do not become infected, but the ship becomes quarantined, you'll have a very unpleasant time in your small cabin.

With Other Conditions

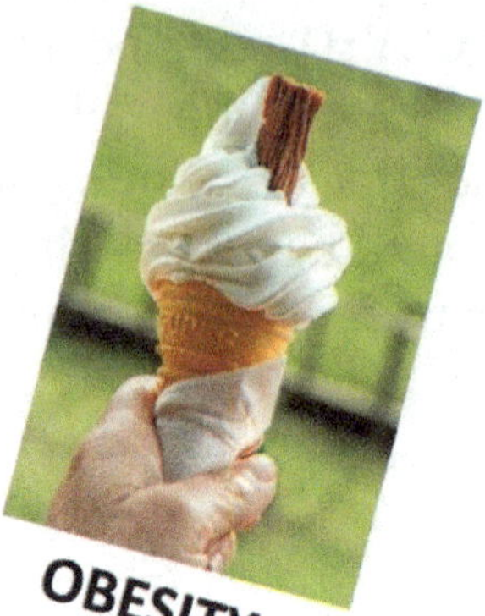

OBESITY

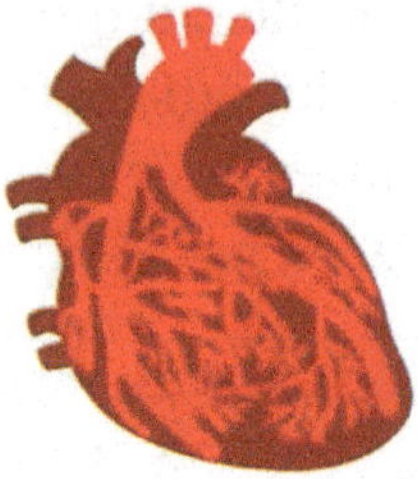

HEART PROBLEMS

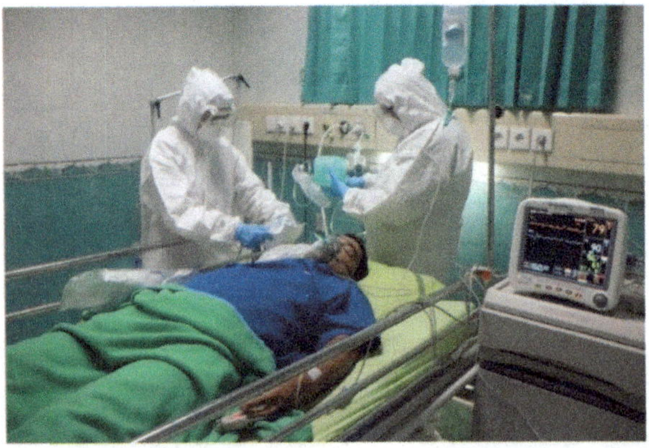

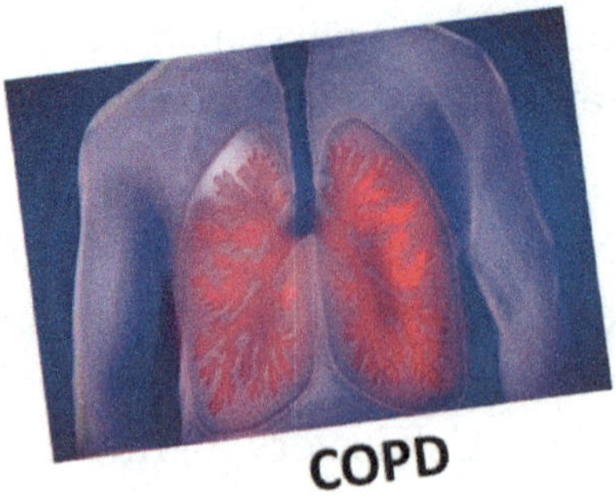

COPD

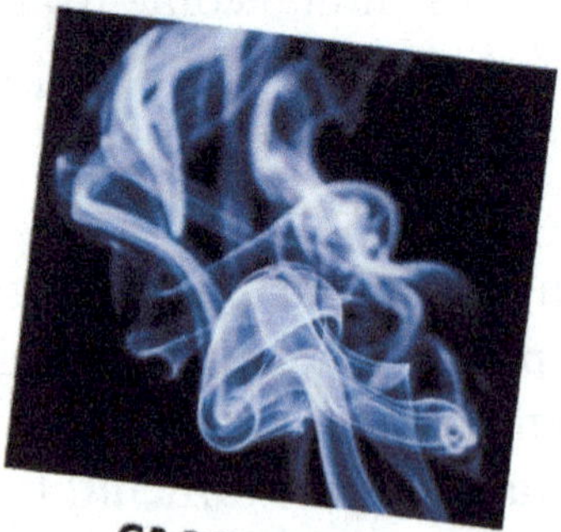

SMOKING

I weigh too much—well, I'm overweight. Quite a bit. Is it true that I'm at higher risk of getting really sick if I come down with COVID-19?

Yes, it's true; your risk is higher. On October 6, 2020, the CDC revised its information and recommendations about underlying medical conditions, including overweight and obesity. These conditions are associated with increased risk of severe illness for adults who become ill with COVID-19.

The body mass index (BMI) gives ranges defining normal weight, overweight, and obesity based on how tall you are. Many BMI calculators are on websites, such as the National Institutes of Health: www.nhibi.nih.gov/health/educational/lose_wt//BMI/bmicalc.htm

The higher one's BMI, the higher that person's risk for serious outcomes from COVID-19.

Okay, so being overweight makes me at greater risk of problems if I catch COVID-19. What should I do?

If you can manage to lose some weight, that could help. Other than that, what the CDC says you need to do is exactly what everyone should do:

Follow the basics—wear a mask, wash your hands, and maintain distance.

But the CDC has added two recommendations for people like you who are at *increased risk* if they come down with COVID-19-10: clean and disinfect surfaces you often touch, and avoid all cruise travel and nonessential air travel. It goes back to what we talked about before—making choices based on your risks. If your risks go up, you need to think seriously about narrowing your choices.

And if you have more than one underlying medical condition, the risk goes up. The more medical conditions, the greater the risk for severe illness from COVID-19.

CDC also recommends that you check with your doctor to see if your vaccinations and other preventive services are up to date. Assess your lifestyle, too. Are you physically active? Are you coping adequately with the stress in your life?

https://www.cdc.gov/coronavirus/2019-ncov/need-extra-precautions/other-at-risk-populations.html

Does the CDC say anything about underlying conditions associated with higher risk?

Yes; general advice and some specific advice.

The general advice:

Continue taking your medicines, don't change your treatment plan without talking with your health care provider. Maintain at least a 30-day supply of your prescription and non-prescription medicines. Talk with your health care provider about getting an extra prescription supply.

Don't delay getting emergency care for your underlying condition(s) because of COVID-19; emergency departments have infection prevention plans ready.

Call your health care provider if you have concerns about your underlying condition(s) or if you become ill and think you may have COVID-19. If you need emergency help, call 911 right away.

For people who don't have a health care provider, the CDC recommends contacting the nearest health department or Federally Qualified Health Center (that's a community-based health care provider funded by the federal Health Resources and Services Administration; it provides primary care services in underserved areas).

The specific advice:

Many of the underlying conditions the CDC lists are fairly common. Sometimes these common conditions can be modified by lifestyle changes, medication, or both. That group includes high blood pressure, type 2 diabetes, and obesity/overweight.

In your case, if you're interested in losing weight, it would be a good idea to talk with your doctor about that. If you do lose weight, you will lower your risk of problems if you come down with COVID-19.

And the CDC strongly recommends getting the flu vaccine. The pandemic makes getting a flu vaccine more important than ever. That's especially true for people at high risk from the flu and also for people who are at high risk if they get COVID-19.

According to the CDC, the conditions that put people at increased risk of severe illness if they become ill with COVID-19 are (in alphabetical order, not by level of risk):

- Cancer
- Chronic kidney disease
- Circulatory problems
- COPD (chronic obstructive pulmonary disease)
- Diabetes mellitus (Types 1 and 2)
- Heart conditions, such as heart failure, coronary artery disease, or cardiomyopathies (various heart diseases)
- Obesity (body mass index [BMI] of 30 kg/m^2 or higher
- Pregnancy and recent pregnancy
- Smoking (current and former)

And the conditions the CDC says *might* put adults at increased risk of severe illness:

- Asthma (moderate to severe)
- Cerebrovascular disease (affects blood vessels and blood supply to the brain)
- Children with certain underlying conditions
- Cystic fibrosis
- Down syndrome
- Hypertension (high blood pressure)
- Immunocompromised state (weakened immune system) from organ, blood, or bone marrow transplantation, immune deficiencies, HIV, use of corticosteroids, or use of other immune weakening medicines
- Neurologic conditions, such as dementia
- Liver disease

- Other lung disease (such as pulmonary fibrosis [damaged or scarred lung tissues])
- Overweight (BMI > 25 kg/m^2, but < 30 kg/m^2)
- Sickle cell disease
- Substance use disorder
- Thalassemia (a type of blood disorder)

The CDC plans to update the lists frequently, so if you're interested, check now and then. Here's the URL:

https://www.cdc.gov/coronavirus/2019-ncov/COVID-19-data/investigations-discovery/assessing-risk-factors.html

Is it true that my blood type will affect how serious my illness will be, if I get COVID-19?

A Canadian study published in *Annals of Internal Medicine* found that O and Rh- blood groups were associated with a slightly lower risk for SARS-CoV-2 infection and for severe COVID-19 illness or death. But the study's authors commented that whether this information can be used to influence the prevention or treatment of COVID-19 "remains to be determined."

https://www.acpjournals.org/doi/10.7326/M20-4511

Does a patient's vitamin D level affect how serious COVID-19 will be?

A report published in *JAMA* in January 2021 reviewed some of the published studies on that topic. The upshot: some studies suggest a relationship between vitamin D levels and the severity of COVID-19, but other studies suggest the opposite.

The author did mention that it's important to avoid vitamin D deficiency. She suggested that if the dietary supply of vitamin D is insufficient, a supplement of the recommended daily allowance, 600 to 1000 IU per day, is a "good idea." She added that she didn't want "to leave the impression that diet cannot be sufficient."

COVID-19!

My big family loves big get-togethers. I'm in one of the high-risk groups, so f I join them, what special care should I take?

The CDC has homed in on social get-togethers and family gatherings when people at increased risk are involved. These gatherings require special planning. If you're immunosuppressed because of an organ transplant, for example, even if you're fully vaccinated you probably have a low antibody response.

If you take part, the CDC recommends you follow certain precautions and limit your interactions with others as much as possible.

To the three basic precautions—masks, handwashing, and social distancing—the CDC suggests adding two daily tasks: cleaning and disinfecting frequently touched surfaces—tables, doorknobs, phones, countertops, handles, desks, keyboards, light switches, toilets, faucets, and sinks. If surfaces are dirty, clean them with detergent or soap and water before disinfecting, the CDC says; then disinfect, using an EPA-registered household disinfectant or alcohol.

Monitor your health daily; look for symptoms of COVID-19—fever, cough, shortness of breath.

If you develop symptoms, take your temperature—but *don't* take it within 30 minutes of exercising or after you take acetaminophen or other medications that could lower your temperature. Then follow CDC guidance if you develop symptoms. If you feel sick and suspect COVID-19, contact your health care provider within 24 hours.

As for acetaminophen—most people have no idea how many medications contain acetaminophen. I knew the number must be high, but I was surprised when I found this statement by the FDA: "What you may not realize is that more than 600 medications, both prescription and over the counter (OTC), contain the active ingredient acetaminophen to help relieve pain and reduce fever."

So those are some things you can do—*if* you decide to take the risk of joining big family get-togethers. But think carefully about whether it's something you really want to do. Don't forget, *you're betting your life!*

Someday this COVID-19 tragedy will ease, and things will start opening up again. How should I plan for going out with others, given my increased risk if I get COVID-19?

The CDC site (https://www.cdc.gov/coronavirus/2019-ncov/daily-life-coping/going-out.html) talks about considering your risk level before you decide to go out, and protecting yourself if you do go out. For example, think about avoiding activities if it would be difficult to take protective measures, such as social distancing if your activities will involve many people.

Also think about who will take part in the get-together and for how long. The more people you interact with, and the closer—and longer—the interaction, the higher your risk of getting COVID-19.

If you do take part, continue with preventive measures and avoid people who aren't wearing masks—or ask them to please put on a mask. Exceptions to mask-wearing include children under age 2 and anyone who has trouble breathing, is unconscious, or is incapacitated or otherwise unable to put on or remove the mask without help.

My kidney problems put me at special risk of more serious disease if I get COVID-19. Is there a way of getting together with family safely?

The basics: postpone or cancel the visit, if, in the 14 days before the visit, any family member had symptoms of COVID-19 or was exposed to someone with COVID-19.

Some issues for you to think about in deciding whether to go:

Are you and the others fully vaccinated? How many people will attend? How long will the get-together last? Will it be held indoors or outside? Will you be able to keep a 6-foot distance from others?

And some suggestions: Visit outdoors, if possible; otherwise choose an area that is well ventilated, with windows or doors open; a place large enough for social distancing. Arrange tables and chairs accordingly, with people from the same households grouped together.

Plan activities that allow people to give each other space, such as yard games. Avoid close contact; greet people with a wave and a few words, rather than a hug or elbow bump.

Keep a list of people you were with and the date of the get-together. If someone contracts COVID-19, all attendees should be notified. The list will make contact tracing much easier.

Remind guests to wash or sanitize their hands before serving or eating food and whenever they may have touched something that might have been contaminated by the virus. Use paper towels to dry and have a no-touch trash can available.

Contact with surfaces or shared items can be limited by having everyone supply their own food and drinks, and by cleaning and disinfecting surfaces and shared items between use.

Because I'm at increased risk of problems if I develop COVID-19, I'm wondering how low-risk gatherings differ from high-risk ones. Do you have information on that?

Yes, indeed.

Lowest risk are virtual-only activities, events, and gatherings. For example, Zoom sessions.

The more-risk category includes smaller outdoor and in-person gatherings, where members of different households wear masks, stay at least 6 feet apart, do not share objects, and come from the same local area (community, city, or county). Get-togethers where eating and drinking occur, and therefore masks cannot be worn, greatly increases the risk for this and other gatherings.

Higher risk are medium-sized, in-person gatherings, where people are at least 6 feet apart and come from outside the local area.

The highest risk is large in-person gatherings, where it's hard to maintain 6-foot spacing and attendees travel from outside the area.

I have a child who has diabetes. Is she at special risk if she gets COVID-19?

The CDC website has quite a bit of information about adults, but not much about children. The website does say that children with the following conditions *might be* at increased risk for severe illness: obesity, medical complexity, severe genetic disorders, severe neurologic disorders, inherited metabolic disorders, congenital (since birth) heart disease, diabetes, asthma and other chronic lung disease, and immunosuppression due to malignancy or immune-weakening medications.

What I'd advise, because of your child's possibly higher risks, is to be sure to follow the three basic precautions—masks, handwashing, and distancing. She should be vaccinated if possible. Also, clean and disinfect areas your child is likely to touch—surfaces of furniture in her room, the kitchen, and family room, or wherever she spends time. Do that often. And following the advice about avoiding cruises and nonessential flying would be a good idea.

I've been a smoker for many years. Am I more likely to get COVID-19?

Several studies have reported that smokers are more likely than nonsmokers to get COVID-19.

Data also indicate that if a smoker becomes infected with COVID-19, the disease is more likely to be severe than in a non-smoker.

Evidence indicates that smoking increases levels of a protein normally present in the lung, called ACE2. The spike protein of SARS-CoV-2 virus particles attaches to the ACE2 protein on the cell surface and allows the virus to enter the cell. That's why the lungs are an attractive field for the virus to invade and replicate.

Therefore, this increase in ACE2 in smokers raises the likelihood of becoming infected with a lower infectious dose of virus, and makes the disease much more severe if it occurs.

COVID-19!

I have a toothache. What should I do?

Clearly, dentists need to be physically close to their patients, but just as clearly, you need to have your tooth taken care of!

Given that it's physically impossible for a dental patient to wear a mask, how risky is a dental visit?

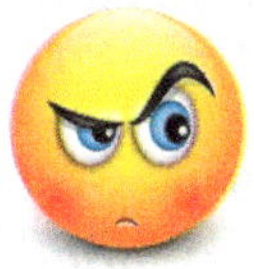

Surprisingly, not very risky at all, according to a study by Dr. Cameron Estrich and colleagues published in *The Journal of the American Dental Association*. Even before vaccines became available, fewer than 1% of U.S. dentists in the study tested positive for COVID-19. That's far below the infection rate of other health professionals. Moreover, according to the study, 99% of dentists routinely use enhanced disinfection practices and other advanced infection-control procedures, as they've done for years.

COVID-19!

I'm pregnant. What should I be doing to protect the two of us?

So far, we haven't enough evidence to know what precautions to recommend. I'm sorry to have to say that so often, but this disease is new to us; the virus is new to us; and we need time to carry out more studies. Also, the vaccine trials excluded pregnant and nursing mothers, because so little was known at that time about possible vaccine risk.

However, the Pfizer/BioNTech and Moderna vaccines have proven to be so safe and effective that it is now recommended that pregnant and nursing mothers be vaccinated. But you should rely on the advice of your obstetrician.

You should, of course, follow the CDC guidelines to minimize your chances of infection.

Even if you become infected with COVID-19 during your pregnancy, the risk that your baby might also be infected is not known, although the limited evidence suggests that the baby is not at serious risk.

Infection of the baby by vertical transmission, that is, from the mother to the fetus, through the placenta, has not been shown, except in a few rare instances. Likewise, infection in the birth canal—the vagina—seems unlikely, because vaginal swabs taken in women known to be infected generally have been negative for the virus.

Infection of the baby soon after birth from environmental virus—what is known as horizontal infection—is also possible; simple isolation procedures appear to prevent it.

I had an organ transplant several years ago, and I'm immunosuppressed. Does that affect my chance of getting COVID-19?

Limited data suggest that someone who's immunosuppressed because of organ transplantation may be more susceptible to infection with SARS-CoV-2.

On the other hand, other limited data suggest that someone who's immunosuppressed and has become infected may be *less likely to have an unfavorable outcome* than someone who is not immunosuppressed. In other words, immunosuppression *may be protective.*

And, yes, this is a bit confusing.

Why could immunosuppression be protective? In a person who is not immunosuppressed, the immune system may overreact in the late stage of a severe infection. This overreaction could cause inflammation of the lungs and other organs, perhaps resulting in a poor outcome. So, patients who are not immunosuppressed are often given immunosuppressive drugs to prevent this overreaction.

We don't know much yet about COVID-19 in this situation. The virus itself and the disease it causes are so new. And that's why we can't answer this question with much confidence.

Far Afield

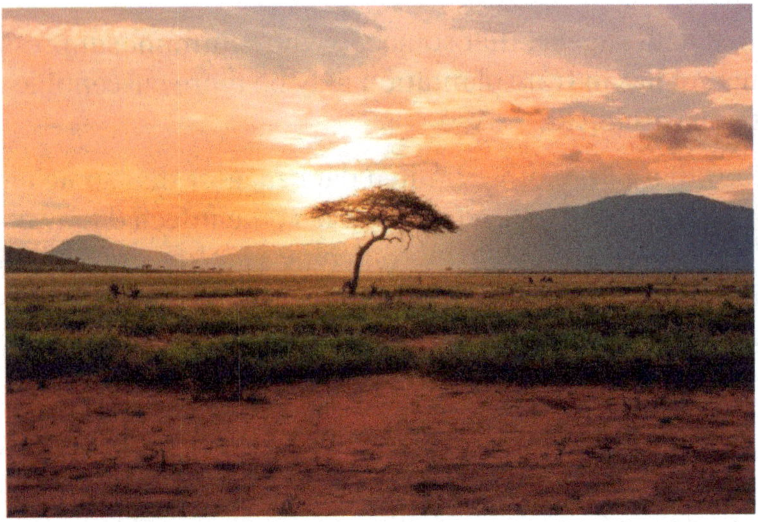

In this section we look at questions from people who have asked for more details about some aspect of COVID-19. We suggest you take a quick look at the questions and see if any topics interest you.

How is stomach flu different from respiratory flu?

There's no disease known medically as stomach flu, although we often hear the term. Stomach flu is described as a combination of nausea, vomiting, and diarrhea.

As for the respiratory disease, the correct name is *influenza,* but flu is often used instead. When we use flu in this book, we always mean the respiratory disease, influenza, rather than a GI—gastrointestinal—condition.

Influenza is caused by the influenza virus. The disease is spread by coughing or sneezing that produces droplets or aerosols. Usually the symptoms last about 5 to 10 days, and can be severe. Those are miserable days for the patient, who may suffer from cough, sore throat, runny nose, general weakness and tiredness, and extreme muscle aches—along with chills and fever.

Interestingly, the worldwide incidence of influenza during the COVID-19 pandemic has been far lower than in previous years. This is because the precautions—masks, social distancing, and hand washing—used by many people for reducing their risk of getting COVID-19 also reduce the risk of catching influenza.

Is this disease worse than the seasonal flu that comes around most years?

COVID-19 is more infective and has a higher fatality rate than seasonal influenza and the influenza of the 1918 pandemic. Even in countries with a lower incidence of COVID-19, the death toll can be much higher from COVID-19 than from seasonal influenza.

COVID-19!

Why so much fuss about COVID-19? Wasn't the flu pandemic about 100 years ago more serious?

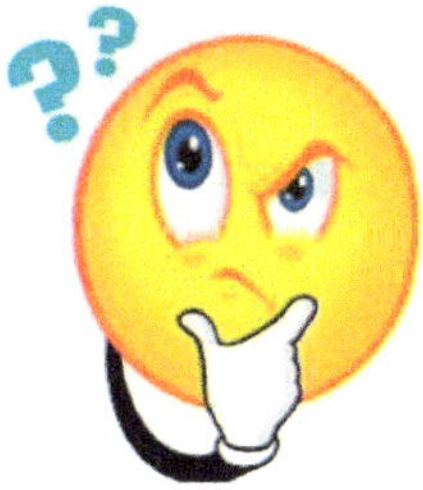

Actually, COVID-19 is more dangerous than the Spanish flu of 1918. There are at least two reasons: the virus that causes COVID-19 is more infective than the influenza virus of 1918, and the fatality rate is higher. In other words, people are more likely to catch COVID-19 and to die from it.

Although you didn't ask, you might be interested in knowing how we measure infectivity during an outbreak, using the term R_0. I know for sure that some of you want to know about the data, so I'll proceed. The rest of you—I don't want to bore you, so . . .

Please just move on to the next question.

****

Scientists use the term R_0, or R0, to describe infectivity during an outbreak. (The term is pronounced either R-*zero* or R-*naught*.)

In brief, R_0 represents the average number of people who will catch the disease from one infected person, in a population that hadn't seen the disease before and hasn't been vaccinated. If R_0 is 3, every case will create three new cases, on average.

This is how that works:

Let's say an infected but asymptomatic person enters a community that is disease-free, and that all inhabitants are susceptible to infection. (The community can be a city, a ship on an extended cruise, a home for elder care, etc.) That one infected person, called patient zero, or the index case, infects three others (R_0 is 3). Each infected person infects three more, and the infections continue:

COVID-19!

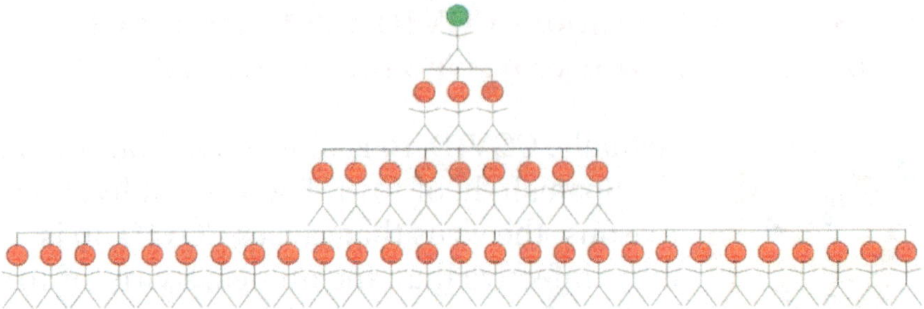

For COVID-19, the period from infection to becoming infectious is about 4 to 5 days on average. So the above increase to 40 cases occurs over about 3 weeks. In another week, it will be over 100 cases. Then 300 cases, and so forth.

If a single case enters a completely susceptible population, the disease can spread to more than a million people in about 2 months. So the pandemic spreads extremely rapidly.

But compare COVID-19 to measles, which has an R_0 of 15 to 18, indicating that measles is a much more contagious disease. Measles also is a deadly disease, but it doesn't cause pandemics. A key reason is that the person infected with measles virus becomes quite sick *before* becoming infectious, and goes to bed early in the disease, having had little or no contact with other people. Also, those other people, such as parents, are probably immune, because measles confers lifelong immunity.

The influenza pandemic of 1918 is similar to the current pandemic, in that no people in the population had any immunity to that virus when it began circulating. The influenza pandemic occurred during World War I, when troops were close to each other (not socially distanced) and were transported by ship from the U.S. to Europe. No vaccine or specific treatment was available, and it wasn't even known that influenza was a viral disease. Even basic knowledge about viruses was quite primitive by today's standard. Also, communication of clinical information was slow by comparison with today, and medical scientists had not developed procedures for clinical trials.

Since then, scientists have learned a great deal about epidemics and pandemics. They now know that if the R_0 is greater than 1, the infection is likely to keep spreading. If it's less than 1, the outbreak will probably die out.

The R_0 alerted some folks early on about trouble ahead with 2019-nCoV9 (the 9 was part of the original name for SARS-CoV-2). *The Atlantic* described this in an article published January 28, 2020, under the headline, The Deceptively Simple Number Sparking Coronavirus Fears, by Ed Yong.

At least six teams of researchers, along with the WHO, have published estimates of R_0 for the new coronavirus. Although these groups used different methods, their results have been consistent, with estimates hovering between 2 and 3. Dr. Salzberger and his team reviewed various estimates of R_0 and settled on a value of 2.5 as of August 2020.

As a reminder, R_0 refers to the average number of people that an infected person will transmit the virus to, assuming the population has no immunity. R_0 changes as the at-risk population changes. For example, as more people recover and develop immunity, or as measures such as masking, social distancing, and quarantines become effective and show results, R_0 decreases. Widespread vaccination with an effective vaccine also decreases R_0. As immunity develops in the population, R_0 decreases, eventually becoming less than 1, when the pandemic dies out.

****

Superspreaders—people who transmit an infectious disease to an unusually large number of other people—seem to play a key role in spreading COVID-19. One infected person can infect many others, typically at large gatherings, indoors or out, when attendees are not wearing masks or not staying at least six feet apart. Studies show that many church gatherings, choir practices, parties at restaurants, and political rallies have turned into superspreading events.

Note that these R_0 rates are based on confirmed cases. Many COVID-19 cases—an unknown number—may be unrecognized. That is, a person may be a carrier—have no symptoms—yet be able to infect others. Carriers may be totally unaware that they have ever been infected. Even with fewer cases, the number of COVID-19 deaths could equal deaths during the 1918 influenza pandemic.

A CDC website lists underlying conditions that put people at increased risk of having a severe illness if they contract COVID-19. The website provides additional information and updates the website content as new information becomes available.

https://www.cdc.gov/coronavirus/2019-ncov/need-extra-precautions/people-with-medical-conditions.html?utm_campaign=20200715_cvd_prv_gal&utm_content=english&utm_medium=email&utm_source=govdelivery

How many people were infected with SARS-CoV, and what kept the outbreak from turning into an epidemic?

In 2003 the coronavirus called SARS-CoV spread from China to several other countries—especially Asia, but also the U.S. and Canada. Confirmed cases totaled 8,096, with 774 deaths. The case fatality rate (CFR) was 9.6%.

The CFR suggests how serious a disease is. Higher rates indicate the likelihood of a severe outcome if you have the disease.

That first coronavirus, SARS-CoV, was different from the current one, the virus that causes COVID-19:

≈ The transmission rate—the rate of new infections in susceptible people—was lower for SARS-CoV

≈ Most new infections came from health care workers who were infected, yet asymptomatic, and had direct contact with patients

And—

≈ *Patients did not shed virus during their incubation period*

This last point is key. The lack of virus shedding with the first coronavirus meant that people who didn't have symptoms weren't passing along the infection. And it may have misled early COVID-19 investigators into believing that the later virus, SARS-CoV-2, might act the same way. That is, they may have decided—incorrectly—that people who didn't have symptoms might not spread the virus.

Another important point: early reports on SARS-CoV-2 *were unclear about whether there was any human-to-human spread at all.* This uncertainty was based in part on experience with the MERS coronavirus. That virus was almost never transmitted between humans; it spread only among camels and from camels to humans.

COVID-19!

We did hear reports from China in January 2020 suggesting human-to-human transmission of COVID-19, but some investigators doubted those reports. China has had a reputation for publishing questionable data.

SARS did not become an epidemic (or pandemic) because it was not transmitted human-to-human until after a person's infection became symptomatic and even then it had a low level of transmissibility.

The SARS outbreak in China, and especially Taiwan, gave the opportunity to develop procedures for preventing spread. Several of the Asian countries used this new knowledge early in the COVID-19 outbreak, and they had far fewer cases and deaths than did other countries.

Why didn't MERS become a pandemic?

Just as COVID-19 and the SARS outbreak of 2003 are caused by coronaviruses, so is Middle Eastern Respiratory Syndrome (MERS). But MERS is largely confined to camels and people who work with camels.

Nearly all camels in Saudi Arabia test positive for the MERS virus. Most infections in humans occur in camel herders and workers who become infected from respiratory droplets released by camels. Human-to-human transmission is rare, unless there's strong exposure—as when health care workers treat MERS patients.

According to the WHO, by November 2019, the MERS virus, MERS-CoV, resulted in 2,494 confirmed cases of MERS and 858 deaths. With the very high case fatality rate of 34.4%—much higher than the rate with COVID-19—how fortunate it was that MERS-CoV couldn't easily transmit disease between humans.

The case fatality rate for MERS probably is more accurate than the rate for COVID-19, because no one carried the MERS virus without showing symptoms.

With limited testing for COVID-19, it's hard to say how many people infected with SARS-CoV-2, the virus that causes COVID-19, show no symptoms. Some reports indicate it may be a very large number.

Do coronaviruses infect other animals?

Yes, there are many different coronaviruses, and they can infect many other animals besides people. The animals we're aware of are bats, whales, gorillas, tigers, camels, pigs, birds, cats, dogs, minks, and mice. But almost certainly, other animals also have undiscovered coronaviruses.

Typically, the natural host—also known as the primary host or reservoir host—shows little or no ill effect from the virus' presence. The animal and the virus have evolved together, and the animal becomes an unharmed carrier. If a natural host does become infected and does harbor the virus, it has no symptoms and is without disease.

Problems can develop if the virus mutates—when the structure of its RNA or DNA undergoes a change. The mutation might make the virus more infective, or less infective; or it might, or might not, make it possible for the virus to infect another animal. If a different kind of animal is infected, the infection can be restricted to the new host, and it can be lethal, but neither possibility is certain.

The virus can undergo a second mutation and jump to a different host, such as a human.

COVID-19!

Where did this coronavirus come from?

Genetics experts have looked into the origin of the three coronaviruses that are dangerous to humans. These virus geneticists have found that the two earlier viruses (SARS-CoV and MERS-CoV) are derived from coronaviruses carried by bats. That's probably true, too, of SARS-CoV-2, the virus that causes COVID-19.

The most likely scenario is that the virus that is carried by bats but causes no disease in bats underwent one or more mutations, enabling it to infect humans. Such "jumping" of a virus of wild animals in which it causes no disease to a new host is known to occur with many other viruses. In some cases, an intermediate host is involved; that is, the virus in its natural host "jumps" to another type of animal, and from that animal to humans.

With SARS-CoV-2, it is not known what the intermediate host might be, although one possibility is the pangolin. This wild animal, which is prized for its scales used in Chinese traditional medicine, is sold in markets including the Wuhan market.

Virus	Primary Host	Intermediate Host	Human Disease
SARS-CoV	Bats	Civets, Raccoon dogs	SARS
MERS-CoV	Bats	Camels	MERS
SARS-CoV-2	Bats?	Unknown	COVID-19

Studies of the viral genes shows that the virus became infective for humans in about late November or early December 2019. By calculating backwards, other researchers also found that first infections with the virus, at a level so low as not to be noticed as unusual, occurred about the same time in people living in Wuhan but not associated with the Wuhan Institute of Virology.

For about 25 years, the virology institute in Wuhan has been actively studying viruses obtained from bats in China. Although the institute has high-level safeguards against viral escape, the possibility that the virus escaped from the virology institute, such as by accidental infection of a laboratory worker, or in laboratory waste, cannot be ruled out.

Presently, either of those two credible hypotheses could account for the origin of SARS-CoV-2, and many other, not-credible hypotheses are common in social media.

Scientists decide between hypotheses based on hard data. Such data have not been available, even to a team from the WHO that visited the institute of virology in Wuhan for the purpose of deciding between the alternate hypotheses. If the Chinese government continues to prevent free access to data from the institute, we'll probably never know for sure how SARS-CoV-2 originated.

I've heard that the virus has been found in sewage. If that's true, could the virus get into our drinking water?

Yes, it's true; investigators in several countries have found viral RNA—traces of the virus—in city wastewater. But they haven't found *infectious* virus.

They've also found that the amount of viral traces in sewage increases a week or more before an outbreak. In fact, some cities now regularly monitor sewage for viral traces. This information can help city health officials predict the need for hospital beds, health care workers, and medical supplies.

To monitor sewage, officials use the RT-PCR test, widely used to test for viral infections in people. What's interesting to me, as a virologist, is that the test is sensitive enough to detect viral RNA in the huge amount of sewage that flows through a city's disposal plants each day. For example, Chicago's Stickney wastewater treatment plant processes about 1.5 billion gallons of wastewater daily.

But remember, the test detects viral RNA, not infectious virus. The possibility that a person could become infected from tap water, even if viral RNA is present, is essentially zero.

What about pets? Can my cat catch the coronavirus?

Yes, a few cats and dogs have been found to carry SARS-CoV-2. Apparently they became infected from contact with an infected person. A tiger at a New York zoo also tested positive, probably infected by a caretaker. Other animals thought to have been infected by humans: hamsters, ferrets, mink, gorillas, and monkeys.

The only humans investigators think may have been infected directly from any of these animals are two mink handlers, but we know very little about that incident.

Many animals, including cats, have their own coronaviruses. When animals are infected with these coronaviruses, the virus usually cannot be transmitted to a different kind of animal, including humans.

It's interesting that animals, unlike people, tend to develop intestinal problems, such as severe diarrhea, from their native coronaviruses, rather than respiratory symptoms.

Why I Wrote This Book

My first phone call came in early March 2020.

"This—coronavirus thing—is it serious? Or are the news media blowing it way out of proportion?"

The caller, a family member we'll call Tom, tends to scoff at press "breaking news" stories, so I wasn't surprised to hear from him.

I answered by emphasizing that this coronavirus news was very serious. What had happened in China, and seemed to be happening in Europe, wasn't caused by politicians or blown up by the media. It was the beginning of an epidemic caused by a virus.

I also told him it resembled, in some ways, the beginning of the 1918-1919 pandemic known as the Spanish flu.

We talked a while, and, when we said goodbye, I hoped I hadn't made Tom more upset than he had been. But I also hoped he realized the gravity of the situation.

A few days later Tom called again. Seems he'd vetted me, checked my answers at the CDC website—that's the Centers for Disease Control and Prevention—and elsewhere, and, maybe somewhat to his surprise, what I'd told him checked out.

Now he had new questions. I had to put him off briefly because another phone call came in. "Hey, Clyde, maybe this is a silly question, but—the wedding is coming up. Should I cancel?"

A cousin was getting married in Wisconsin; the caller lived in New York City. The answer was easy: "Cancel the tickets and stay home."

COVID-19!

Why They Called Me

In addition to being a medical doctor, I'm a virologist by training and experience. Wrote a virology textbook, *An Introduction to Virology*, years ago; taught virology courses to college students and medical students; and held a professorship in microbiology at Rush Medical School in Chicago.

And I've been around long enough to have been involved with viral epidemics on a personal level.

That includes some bleak times and some truly upsetting memories. I've treated patients during several seasonal influenza outbreaks, but one I remember was especially bad. Several times I rushed out on a house call and arrived within minutes—only to be told by a tearful family member that their loved one had died, just moments before. I was a very young doctor and the experience was extremely distressing.

History: The Spanish Flu, 1918

About 20 years ago, a paper I'd written on the 1918 influenza pandemic, the Spanish flu, "Will The Next Outbreak Spell Disaster?" was the cover story in *Laboratory Medicine*. (No, I wasn't around in 1918; I'm not that old!) The issue's cover depicted an ominous scene: a ship, symbolizing the *Titanic*, heading for an iceberg.

Research Gate notified me early in April (2020) that hits on my article were spiking. Perhaps readers were seeing similarities between the 1918 pandemic and the current one.

Similarities do exist; but so do differences.

- The 1918 disease produced an overwhelming, often deadly, pneumonia in many patients, just as COVID-19 can. Pneumonia often destroys the lungs, making breathing impossible, even with ventilator help.

- A huge difference with the current pandemic is the knowledge level. Little was known about any viruses in 1918. It wasn't until 1933 that scientists discovered that the 1918 pandemic wasn't a bacterial disease; it was caused by a virus. Today we know far more about viruses and pandemics.
- Supportive care is much better now. And we have antibiotics to treat secondary bacterial infections (although antibiotics have no effect on the viral infection). Modern medical care is surely saving more lives than would have occurred if COVID-19 had hit in 1918.
- As this pandemic continues, scientific studies worldwide are being published in top medical and scientific journals. Before now it took almost a year to publish scientific articles; today important articles can appear in journals within a few weeks. Medical scientists can now access authoritative information on the internet within minutes and apply it to help patients and save lives.
- On the downside, the internet has also made it possible for misinformation, crazy conspiracy theories, and even downright lies to spread to a public with many people who cannot tell truth from fiction. A goal of this book is to help dispel some of the misinformation.

Ominous Thoughts

As I turned my thoughts back to the present pandemic, I had an ominous feeling. I sensed that something truly frightening was developing. I worried. What if mutants—variants—emerged? And I worried that what Tom had called the "coronavirus thing" could escalate into a pandemic every bit as deadly as the Spanish flu—the most severe pandemic in recent history—or one even more deadly.

Yet skepticism prevailed, even among some doctors. A man who briefly shared an elevator in mid-March with my wife, Barbara, asked her what she thought about the coronavirus disease. "It's nothing, right?" he said. "My brother is an emergency room doctor here in Fort Lauderdale, and he says he's not seeing any coronavirus cases. Just a few patients with the usual flu. He says the new virus is nothing more than the flu."

As Barbara got out of the elevator, she said, "I don't agree. And my husband, who's an MD virologist, thinks it's very serious." If that man was seeking reassurance, he didn't get it.

The World Health Organization (WHO) eventually helped banish some skepticism on March 11, 2020, declaring the outbreak of COVID-19 a pandemic.

Full Disclosure

About my background: I've worked directly with many viruses, published dozens of research papers, and wrote a popular virology textbook. But I've had no direct laboratory experience with SARS-CoV-2, the virus that causes COVID-19. Of course, until December 2019, no one else had either.

So, instead of relying on laboratory experience, I've researched the literature to get up to speed and keep up. I know how to assess credibility of information and sort out scientific fact from pseudoscience—and there's a lot of that on the web—and from comments on TV and in the press by reporters and politicians. I needed to ensure that this book has the latest reliable information about SARS-CoV-2 and COVID-19.

My Qualifications

So, who am I? You haven't seen me on news stations, wearing a television-blue shirt, and being introduced as a renowned researcher; or clad in a white coat, stethoscope dangling, being presented as a famous medical practitioner. That's not me.

What I am is an MD virologist with a broad background, and the seasoned perspective that goes with it.

My family tells me that what's probably even more important, where writing books is concerned, is that they think I have a knack for teaching and for explaining things, using words and concepts that people can understand. And for going beyond just conveying information. At least that's what they tell me.

Let me explain something that might be helpful. Early in our careers, we doctors learn to appreciate the many differences in peoples' personalities. We learn that helping some people may mean going beyond just answering questions about their condition. It often also means addressing underlying concerns and offering suggestions and reassurance.

More Calls, More Questions

Calls continue to come in. The callers are friends, relatives, and neighbors, people I know well and care about. They are upset, as we all are.

Some callers are skeptical about the COVID-19 information they're getting from their usual sources. They're frustrated by conflicting information coming from TV, blogs, social media, and print media. And they're frustrated for good reason. They want to make up their own mind, and they want solid data. They want to rely for the most part on a single source of information—but *timely* information—the kind we'll continue to provide with our website updates.

Staying Current

We, too, have been frustrated, but for a different reason. Sometimes we've added detailed new information to our draft, then found a day or two later that what we wrote had just become obsolete.

What had happened? A new study had just come out with good data, or a medical organization had changed its definition of a key term, or a government agency had revised its recommendations. We need to share the new information with you, but we finally faced the fact that we had to publish knowing that the next updates will need to be on our website.

That website for periodic updates is:

www.covid-19faqbook.com.

Most of the questions and answers in this book focus on viruses and general aspects of the pandemic. Some questions involve clinical situations, and for these we provide general comments, and, in some cases, references. If these situations apply to you or your family, it's essential for you to reach out to your physician or your child's pediatrician for personal medical guidance.

Acknowledgements

It is my great honor and pleasure to thank the many people who helped in writing this book. First, early in 2020, queries came from family members about the developing pandemic, showing me the need for a book on COVID-19 that would answer their many questions. (The answers, however, were just beginning to become known to the medical community—and, in fact, many "answers" were later debunked and replaced as new data became available.) Questions from our family and friends kept coming during the writing of the book, as the pandemic unfolded.

I cannot thank enough the many beta readers who saw the early drafts. Their comments were priceless in helping guide the book's development. Some beta readers posed questions to be added and answered, others performed detailed and very helpful editing, and all gave us ample encouragement to keep going.

My heartfelt thanks go to my immediate family members Brian, Ken, and Violet Goodheart; and to additional family members Nancy Hartley, Larry McDonald, and Evert Bergquist. Many thanks also to fellow writers Fern Brown, and Ann-Louise Truschel (Ann-Louise also did a great job of copyediting the early draft).

I also called upon fellow members of the American Medical Writers Association (AMWA) for their input. Two members—Judy Stone, MD and Larry Lynam, DSc—have such a deep knowledge of COVID-19 that I was left wondering why they weren't writing their own Covid book! Thanks also to fellow AMWA members Amanda Mao, PhD; Lynne Schneider, PhD; Shara Pantry, PhD; and Stanley Sack, MD.

And thanks to our friends Betty Kohlberg and Anthony ("Bert") Bertolini, and Joseph Williams, David Mulhern, and Larry

Folgo, who commented on the book from the all-important perspective of the typical reader.

The wonderful cartoon and pictures of the boy in a bubble and the girl in a socially distanced skirt are creations of the very talented artist, David Miller, Kuala Lumpur, Malaysia. Thanks, David!

Family, medical and scientific experts, other beta readers, and our artist–many, many thanks to you all.

But I cannot begin to thank enough my wonderful wife, Barbara. After my many pleadings, she finally agreed to share authorship and made a tremendous difference, with her well-honed writing and editorial inputs, development of the Glossary, discussions, and continued encouragement.

Last, but by far not the least, I owe a huge debt of gratitude to Northwestern University for a fine education. Not only did I earn my four degrees there, but best of all, I met Barbara. That was in a laboratory for Comparative Anatomy (I was the instructor, she was a student). One thing led to another, and we got married.

Many thanks to all of you!

Clyde R. Goodheart, MD, MBA, MS, BS

Index to Questions

COVID-19!

COVID-19!

Glossary

Terms are defined in the context of the SARS-CoV-2 pandemic. Some words defined here do not appear elsewhere in the book.

Most words are defined in one paragraph. For some words, additional details follow the basic definition in a new paragraph.

Acute respiratory distress syndrome (ARDS): a potentially fatal condition in which fluid builds up in the tiny elastic air sacs (alveoli) in the lungs, resulting in severe shortness of breath and insufficient oxygen supply to body tissues

To function normally, the tissues and organs of the body need a constant supply of oxygen. Normally, oxygen from the air we breathe is carried in the bloodstream from the lungs to the body tissues and organs, and carbon dioxide, a waste product, is carried back to the lungs for removal from the body. In ARDS, fluid buildup in the alveoli prevents the lungs from adequately filling with air, and the lungs can no longer deliver enough oxygen to the tissues.

Aerosol: a suspension of tiny solid or liquid particles in air (cigarette smoke—often called *vapor*—is an example); similar to a droplet, but smaller, measuring less than 5 micrometers (µm); a common vehicle for spreading SARS-CoV-2; *see also* Droplet

Antibody: a protective protein the immune system produces in response to a foreign body (antigen), such as a virus;

antibodies latch onto antigens, and both are removed from the body; *see also* Neutralizing antibody

Antibody test (also known as serology test or blood test); a laboratory procedure that uses a blood sample to check for *previous* COVID-19 infection by identifying SARS-CoV-2 antibodies; if antibodies against coronavirus are present, it means that the person has been infected but probably is no longer infectious; that is, the disease has run its course and the patient no longer has COVID-19; if antibodies are *not* present, it does not necessarily mean that the person has not had COVID-19, because false-negative results can occur; it may be necessary to repeat the test if antibodies are not found

Antigen: any foreign substance, such as a virus, that causes the immune system to produce antibodies; if the antibodies connect with antigens, both are removed from the body

Antigen test (rapid diagnostic test): a diagnostic test that uses a sample taken from the patient's nose or throat to check for existing SARS-CoV-2 infections; antigen tests are more rapid than molecular tests but are more likely to miss an active infection (that is, they carry a higher risk of false-negative test results, so they're more likely to yield a negative test result in someone who actually has COVID-19); following up with a molecular test may be indicated

Asymptomatic: without symptoms; showing no signs of disease

A person can be without symptoms in the early stages of COVID-19, and some infected people never develop symptoms. People who are infected but without symptoms can have *false-negative* test results, that is, results that indicate, incorrectly, that they are not infected. These people believe themselves COVID-19-free, so they don't self-isolate; unfortunately, that may not be true, so they may infect others.

At-home collection tests: the patient collects a saliva sample or a nasal-swab sample and sends it to a laboratory for analysis

Basic reproductive number (or ratio) (R_0) (pronounced R-*zero* or *R-naught)*: the number of people an infected person will, on average, infect in a susceptible population; an important indication of how easily a disease is likely to spread in a community

When the basic reproductive number is *less than* 1 ($R_0 < 1$), each person infected, on average, passes along the infection to less than one new person. Thus, an outbreak is likely to die out. If the basic reproductive number is *greater than* one ($R_0 > 1$), the virus can invade the susceptible population.

Case fatality rate (CFR): a ratio that indicates the risk of death from a contagious disease; calculated by dividing the number of deaths by the number of cases in a given time period; factors influencing the CFR are the speed at which cases are diagnosed and the capacity of the health system (*see also* Mortality rate)

Clinical disease: a disease that has recognizable clinical signs and symptoms, as distinct from a subclinical illness, which lacks detectable signs and symptoms. Diabetes, for example, can be a subclinical disease for some years before becoming a clinical disease

Clinical trial: A research study; the gold-standard study is a randomized, placebo-controlled, double-blind trial, with participants assigned by chance to one of two (or more)

unidentified groups to eliminate bias; the goal of the study is to evaluate the effects of intervention on outcomes, such as curing the disease, controlling symptoms, or prolonging life

Test group: study participants who receive the experimental intervention, such as a new drug

Control group: study participants who receive either a placebo or standard care

Placebo-controlled study: a study in which one group of participants receives an inactive substance, and the other group or groups receive the treatment being tested (usually a drug or vaccine)

Double-blind study: a study in which neither the investigator nor the participant knows who is in the test group and who is in the control group until the trial is over

Randomized study: a study whose participants are selected by chance to be in test or control groups

Close contact: being within six feet of an infected person or persons for a *cumulative* total of 15 minutes or more during a 24-hour period; the period starts two days before the illness began for the infected person (or, for asymptomatic patients, two days before the test specimen was collected) and ends when the patient is isolated

Note that individual exposures totaling 15 minutes during 24 hours, such as three 5-minute exposures, are now considered close contact. Previously, close contact was defined as being within six feet of an infected person for 15 minutes or more. The definition was changed on October 21, 2020, after studies suggested that greater exposure is associated with higher risk, even if the exposure occurs during scattered time periods

Factors epidemiologists consider in defining close contact:

- Proximity (closer distance likely increases exposure risk)
- Duration of exposure (longer exposure probably increases exposure risk)
- Presence or absence of symptoms (the time around symptom onset is associated with the highest levels of viral shedding—release from the body of viral particles that may or may not be infectious)
- Likelihood that respiratory aerosols were generated, for example, through coughing, sneezing, shouting, or singing
- Presence or absence of other environmental factors, for example, crowding, adequate ventilation, indoor vs. outdoor exposure

Community spread (community transmission): circulation of an infectious disease among people in a given area when the mode of infection is unknown; that is, the people who became infected had no known contact with a diagnosed individual and hadn't traveled recently to an area of active disease

Confirmed positive case: a case verified by a laboratory test for COVID-19 or by the provider's documentation that the individual has COVID-19; *see also* Presumptive positive case

Contact tracing: identifying people who may have been in contact with someone who has COVID-19; people identified through contact tracing as possibly being infectious are monitored; often they decide to self-quarantine to help control spread of the disease

Contactless: without contact; a tool to help prevent spread of COVID-19; examples of contactless behavior: retailers leaving deliveries at a customer's front door, or loading customers' purchases into a car trunk

Contagious disease: an illness easily transmitted between people; the illness can spread rapidly from person to person 1) by physical contact (as in touching an infected person or object and then touching the eyes, nose, or mouth, thus allowing the organism to enter the body); or by contact with blood or body fluids of an infected person (as in kissing, tending to a wound, or sexual contact); or 2) by inhaling a droplet or aerosol when an infected person breathes, coughs, sneezes, or talks; *see also* Direct contact transmission and Indirect contact transmission

Containment area: a zone with limited access, created to help prevent an outbreak from spreading

Coronavirus (CoV): a member of the *Coronaviridae* family of viruses; SARS-CoV-2 is the coronavirus that causes COVID-19; the six other identified members of the family currently known to infect people and the diseases they cause are SARS-CoV (severe acute respiratory syndrome) and MERS-CoV (Middle East respiratory syndrome), along with four of the more than 200 other viruses that cause the common cold

Often it's said that the coronaviruses were so named because the spikes on their surface resemble the top of a crown. Instead, they are named for their resemblance to the solar corona—the sun's crown.

Anonymous. Coronaviruses. *Nature*. 1968;220:650.

COVID-19!

COVID-19: coronavirus disease 2019 (from co *corona,* vi *virus,* d *disease)*, the disease at the heart of the current pandemic; the organism causing COVID-19 is SARS-CoV-2 (severe acute respiratory syndrome coronavirus 2), first detected in December 2019

Cross-reaction: an antigen-antibody reaction, usually relatively weak, to a pathogen; the reaction results from a previous antigen-antibody reaction to an unrelated pathogen

It is possible that infection with a virus not necessarily related to SARS-CoV-2 could result in at least partial protection against SARS-CoV-2 infection. Such partial protection, a cross-reaction, is known to occur in some viral infections. For example, some cases of COVID-19 may have been milder than expected because the patient previously had a common cold caused by one of the common-cold coronaviruses, and later, when infected with SARS-CoV-2, developed a cross-reaction that provided partial protection.

Diagnostic test: a test to determine if someone is infected with SARS-CoV-2; *see also* Tests for COVID-19

Diagnostic tests for coronavirus: procedures that look for evidence of coronavirus; these include antigen tests and molecular tests (such as RT-PCR); usually diagnostic tests are performed on nasal or throat-swab samples, but a few use saliva samples; *see also* Diagnostic tests for COVID-19

Diagnostic tests for COVID-19: these diagnostic tests are of two types; *molecular tests,* such as RT-PCR tests, detecting the virus's genetic material, and *antigen tests,* detecting specific proteins on the virus's surface; both can detect SARS-CoV-2 specifically, not just coronaviruses as a group; most diagnostic tests use samples taken by nasal or throat swab, but some molecular tests use saliva samples

When we speak of molecular tests detecting a virus's *genetic material,* we're referring to detecting the RNA of a virus or the DNA of a virus. All coronaviruses are RNA viruses, so in this book we say, "detecting the virus's RNA."

Direct contact transmission: the spread of viral disease by direct physical contact between the blood or body fluids of an infected person and a susceptible person; examples include kissing, sexual contact, touching, and contact with oral secretions or with wounds or sores on the body

Disease: any harmful deviation from the normal structural or functional state of an organism, generally associated with certain signs and symptoms and differing in nature from physical injury. A diseased organism commonly exhibits signs or symptoms indicative of its abnormal state.

Disease transmission: diseases such as COVID-19 are spread either of two ways: by *direct contact transmission,* involving physical contact between someone who is infected and someone who is susceptible; or by *indirect contact transmission,* entailing spread through droplets or globules emitted when an infected person coughs or sneezes; *see also* Direct contact transmission and Indirect contact transmission

Drive-thru testing: a procedure performed at a testing station; in a typical example, the patient stays in the car and a health care worker standing outside wearing protective gear reaches through an open car window and uses a swab to obtain a nasal sample

Droplet: a relatively large bit of mucus or saliva, produced by sneezing, coughing, singing, or talking; some researchers estimate the size of droplets as between 5 and 100 μm (for reference, an average human hair is about 75 μm in diameter); larger droplets—known as globules—fall faster than they can evaporate and usually travel less than 6 feet before falling to the ground

Droplet transmission: the spreading of virus particles by the release of mucus or saliva from the mouth; when someone talks, droplets released from the mouth travel a short distance (less than 6 feet), but sneezes, coughs, or singing can propel droplets as far as 25 feet

Endemic: pertaining to a persistent, usually relatively low level of disease cases in a community or geographic area

Epidemic: a sudden widespread, very steep increase in the number of cases of a specific infectious disease

Epidemic curve: a characteristic appearance of a line in a graph or chart, showing the incidence of new cases of a specific disease, over time, after the first diagnosis

Epidemiology: a branch of medical science involved in the incidence, distribution, analysis, and control of infectious diseases

Essential business: an establishment or service critically important in everyday living; examples include hospitals, clinics, grocery stores, banks, pharmacies, gas stations, transportation services

Exposure: contact with a person who has a communicable disease

False-positive test result: a result on a viral test incorrectly identifying someone as being infected; possible consequences are unnecessary quarantine and involvement in contact tracing

False-negative test result: a false-negative result can be more serious than a false-positive result; infected people wrongly believed to be virus-free aren't quarantined and may infect others

Fatality rate: ***see*** **Case fatality rate**

First responder: in a medical situation, a person certified to provide emergency medical care until more highly trained medical personnel arrive

Flattening the curve: the "curve" depicts the number of people expected to contract COVID-19 during a given period; "flattening the curve" means slowing the rate of new infections; the hope is that spreading the number of new infections over a longer period will avoid overburdening the health care system

https://www.livescience.com/coronavirus-flatten-the-curve.html

Forehead thermometer: a device that measures the temperature of the forehead by hovering near it or barely touching it

Fully vaccinated: at least two weeks after the two injections of the Pfizer/BioNTech or Moderna vaccines or the one Johnson & Johnson vaccine

Globule: a relatively large mass of mucus or saliva emitted from a person's mouth or nose while talking, sneezing, coughing, or sneezing; to summarize, here's how suspensions of solid or liquid particles in air are classified by size: aerosol, less than 5 micrometers (μm); droplet: 5 to 100 μm; globule, more than 100 μm

Health care provider: a person who is licensed, certified, registered, or otherwise authorized by state law to provide medical care in the defined scope of practice; examples include doctor of medicine or osteopathy, podiatrist, dentist, chiropractor, clinical psychologist, optometrist, physician assistant, nurse practitioner, nurse-midwife, and clinical social worker

Herd immunity (community immunity): a degree of resistance to the spread of COVID-19; herd immunity occurs when many people in a community have become immune, and the rate of new infections has slowed because the virus has too few new hosts

People can develop immunity by forming antibodies through vaccination or by having the disease. The percentage of people needed to be vaccinated or infected for immunity to develop varies by disease. With measles, it's been estimated that about 83% to 94% of the population must be vaccinated or have had measles for herd immunity to occur. With SARS-CoV-2, estimates are that at least 70% of the population must have antibodies for herd immunity; that's a lower percentage, but immunity to SARS-CoV-2 may last only a few months in a given person, although that estimate may change as we gain more information.

Horizontal transmission: spread of an infectious agent by close contact with other susceptible individuals, rather than through the placenta to an unborn child; *also see* Vertical transmission

Hydroxychloroquine: an oral medication used to treat malaria, rheumatoid arthritis, and lupus; some have promoted it as a treatment for COVID-19, but studies have shown no benefit; moreover, hydroxychloroquine carries substantial risk in the group of people most vulnerable to SARS-CoV-2

Immune surveillance: the immune system's ongoing monitoring of the body to detect, inactivate, or destroy foreign substances, damaged tissues, or dead cells

Immunity: the body's acquired ability to defend against attack by specific infectious agents or certain other substances; immunity may develop from being infected or from being vaccinated

Immunocompromised: having a weakened immune system and therefore being less able to fight infections and other diseases; conditions associated with immunocompromise include HIV, lymphoma, and several other diseases

Immunosuppression: curtailment of the immune system; a state in which the immune system does not function normally because of health conditions unrelated to COVID-19; immunosuppression can result from anticancer medications and other drug treatments; people who are immunosuppressed are at increased risk of being infected by SARS-CoV-2, but a new study indicates that people who are immunosuppressed are not at greater risk of severe disease, as had been thought

https://www.jhsph.edu/news/news-releases/2021/covid-19-outcomes-for-patients-on-immunosuppressive-drugs-on-par-with-non-immunosuppressed-patients.html#:~:text=Estimates%20suggest%20that%20there%20are,spread%20unchecked%20in%20the%20body.

Incubation period: the time between an individual's exposure to a virus and the time the first symptoms of infection appear; with COVID-19, the incubation period is four to five days; people are most infectious from a few days before symptoms begin until a few days after symptoms appear

Index case: the first documented case of a communicable disease within a population

Index patient: the first person identified as having a disease when an outbreak develops; the term is interchangeable with *patient zero*

Indirect contact transmission: the spread of infectious diseases through droplets or aerosols emitted when an infected person talks, coughs or sneezes

Susceptible people become infected when they inhale the secretions, or when the secretions land in, or close to, their eyes, mouth, or nose. Alternatively, infection can occur when secretions land on objects, such as tables and doorknobs, and healthy people touch the contaminated surfaces, then touch their eyes, mouth, or nose, allowing the viruses to enter the body.

Infectious: refers to the spread of an infection, or the likelihood of spreading, or the ability to spread an infection; example: "the patient is still infectious, thus can spread the disease to others"

Infectious disease: a disorder that is transmitted by microorganisms in air or water—bacteria, viruses, parasites, or fungi; some infectious diseases can be spread, directly or indirectly, from one person to another; *see also* Disease transmission; *see also* Contagious disease

Infectious dose: the least amount of infectious material, such as the number of virus particles, that usually produces an infection

Infective: producing, or capable of producing, an infection; refers to the *cause* of an infection

Intensivist: a physician who specializes in treating patients in intensive care or in intensive care units

International Committee on Taxonomy of Viruses (ICTV): an organization that names and classifies newly discovered viruses; the ICTV uses a template to describe, name, and classify the viruses that affect living organisms; ICTV also maintains an information database that is open to the public

Isolation: a procedure for 1) a person who has symptoms of COVID-19, or 2) a person who has tested positive for infection with SARS-CoV-2, the virus that causes COVID-19; until it is safe to be around others, a person in isolation stays alone at home in a sick room (or stays in a hotel or motel) and uses a separate bathroom, if one is available

Isolation is *not* the same as quarantine. A person under quarantine *may have been infected* because of contact with someone who has COVID-19. In contrast, a person in isolation is *known to have been—or highly likely to have been—infected* and is kept away from others, even in the home.

A person in isolation needs to:

- Monitor any symptoms
- Seek emergency medical care immediately if a warning sign develops—such as trouble breathing
- Avoid contact with others, including pets
- Avoid sharing personal household items, such as cups, towels, and utensils

K-12 online instruction: a type of virtual schooling developed in the 1990s; instruction is delivered through technology to students who are separated from their schools and their teachers; formal virtual schools have been established across the country for general education and special education; levels covered include kindergarten through 12th grade

Elementary school students in the program typically need to have their parents involved, but students at middle school and high school often work independently and take part in group and individualized learning programs by means of email, telephone, or video. Usually it's not necessary for students and teachers to be online at the same time, thereby giving students flexibility as to when and where they take part.

K-12 online and blended instruction: a type of K-12 online instruction that includes some face-to-face instruction; *see also* K-12 online instruction

LAMP test: a molecular test to detect SARS-CoV-2; the first such diagnostic test to be used at home, with results available at home in about 30 minutes; the LAMP test was recently granted emergency use authorization (EUA) by FDA

The LAMP test is based on loop-mediated isothermal amplification (LAMP), a technology that is similar to the gold-standard PCR technology. The LAMP test is easier to use than PCR tests, and offers a rapid, portable alternative to traditional testing.

Lockdown: an emergency measure restricting people from certain areas or physically distancing them from others by encouraging or requiring them to stay home; the goal is to control exposure or prevent disease transmission; lockdowns can help slow COVID-19 transmission, but can have a negative economic impact and a negative psychological and social impact as well

MERS-CoV (Middle-East respiratory syndrome coronavirus): this virus causes a disease (MERS) that occurs only in the Middle East, almost exclusively in Saudi Arabia; the transmission rate (R_0) between people is less than 1 (the rate would have to be higher than 1 to sustain the disease in the population); in almost all cases people acquire the disease directly from camels when camels emit droplets during coughing or sneezing; since September 2012, the WHO has been notified of 2,494 cases, with 858 deaths (for a case fatality rate of 34.4%)

Minimal infectious dose: the smallest quantity of infectious material, such as virus particles, that, on average, produces infection in one-half of people exposed

Molecular test: highly accurate diagnostic tests that check for existing COVID-19 infection, usually using a sample from the patient's nose or throat (a few tests use saliva); examples are: RT-PCR test, LAMP test, and the nucleic acid amplification test (NAAT)

Mortality rate: a ratio that indicates the number of deaths in a given period of time in a population; *see also* Fatality rate

Multigenerational household: a unit of three or more generations living together, typically grandparents, parents, and children

Mutation: a change in the genetic code of a virus or organism that is passed on unchanged to its descendants; a mutation can make the organism or virus better adapted to its host or environment, or the mutation can be detrimental, in which case the descendants may die out over succeeding generations

National emergency: an emergency state that allows a government to take measures not normally permitted; can occur during a national disaster, epidemic, pandemic, or other threatening situation

Natural host (of a virus): a type (species) of animal that shows no signs of disease when infected by the virus in question; disease occurs only when a mutation in the circulating virus allows it to infect another type of animal; evidence suggests that bats, a common host of SARS-CoV-2, carried the virus asymptomatically before a mutation enabled SARS-CoV-2 to infect humans

N95 mask (N95 respirator): a type of personal protective equipment some health care workers wear; it forms a tight seal around the nose and mouth; an N95 mask resembles a surgical mask but is a respirator that filters out at least 95% of particles in the air

The N95 mask requires a 20-minute "fit test," and doesn't adequately protect people who have facial hair. At this writing (08/20/2020) the CDC does not recommend N95 respirators for public use.

Neutralizing antibody: an antibody that blocks (neutralizes) the infectivity of a virus

Nosocomial infection: an infection acquired in a hospital or other health care facility

Novel coronavirus (nCoV): a temporary name given to a new coronavirus by the first researchers who identify and describe it; later the new coronavirus is officially named by the International Committee on Taxonomy of Viruses

Outbreak: a sudden increase in cases of an infectious disease; the term is often used to describe an occurrence similar to an epidemic but smaller in scale and limited in area

COVID-19!

Pandemic: a widespread outbreak of an infectious disease, covering a greater area than an epidemic and affecting a large proportion of the world's population

Patient zero: the first person identified as having a disease when an outbreak develops; the term is interchangeable with *index patient*

PCR test (polymerase chain reaction test): a laboratory procedure that detects the genetic material of a virus; to perform the test, a health care worker collects saliva or fluid from a patient's nose or throat

Person-to-person transmission: the spread of a virus among people through physical contact or coughing and sneezing, as opposed to contact with animals or with contaminated objects or surfaces

Physical distancing: avoiding close contact with others; typically, the recommended distance is at least six feet

Placebo: an inactive substance used as a control in a clinical trial; usually a tablet, pill, or vial of liquid that looks like the active drug used in the study

PPE: personal protective equipment; special clothing or gear, such as gowns, face shields, and gloves, to help health care workers guard against exposure to infectious diseases

Presymptomatic: pertaining to the early stage of infection, before symptoms develop

Probable COVID-19 case: a term used to describe a person as meeting clinical *and* epidemiologic evidence of COVID-19, but without confirmatory laboratory evidence

Prodrome: the period when someone who is infected may feel not quite normal but hasn't yet developed definitive symptoms; the person isn't aware of being infected but may be infectious

PUI: person under investigation; someone who may have COVID-19

Quarantine: a noun or verb pertaining to seclusion of someone who is asymptomatic but has been—or is believed to have been—in close contact with a person who has COVID-19; the goal is to protect others from possible exposure in case the person under quarantine later tests positive for the disease; an exception: someone who has had COVID-19 within three months before the close contact occurred *does not* need to quarantine; quarantine may be voluntary or it may be ordered by federal, state, or local public health authorities

People under quarantine need to stay home until 10 days after their last contact with an infected person, checking their temperature twice a day and watching for symptoms of COVID-19: *see also* Close contact

According to a recent article in *Science*, "the word 'quarantine' is derived from the word for '40 days,' from an old Venetian dialect—the period for which incoming ships had to anchor in the harbor to avoid bringing in the plague," in the European Middle Ages during the Black Death pandemic. Other sources suggest that the Venetian word was derived from the early French word "*quarantaine*"—"period of 40 days"—from the still earlier word "*quarante*"—meaning "forty," which, in turn, came from the Latin word for forty, "*quadraginta*."

Remdesivir: an investigational antiviral drug given intravenously; developed for treating Ebola, remdesivir inhibits viral replication; although previously considered by some as a promising drug for treating COVID-19, recent data do not support this use

Replication: The method by which new copies of a virus are made (cell division is not an option, because viruses aren't cells)

During replication, a virus invades a host cell and turns the cell into a "factory" for making more viruses—copies of itself. It does so by first attaching itself to the host cell and inserting its genetic material—RNA—into the cell's machinery. The RNA serves as instructions to the host cell. The host cell responds by producing the various parts of the virus, assembling the parts, and releasing new viruses to the outside. With most viruses, infected cells die after the new viruses are released.

Reproductive number: *see* Basic reproductive number

Respirator: 1) a device worn over the mouth and nose or over the entire face; protects against inhaling dangerous substances, such as particles that may carry the SARS-CoV-2 virus; 2) a device that helps people breathe when they cannot breathe naturally

Risk: the chance that a specified event will happen; the event can range from becoming infected with SARS-CoV-2 to being hit by lightning

Risk is expressed several ways, including "the chance of (the problem developing) is 21%;" or "21 out of 100 people will (develop the problem);" or "about one-fifth of the group will (develop the problem)."

R_0: the average number of people who will catch COVID-19 from one infected person in a population that initially had no previous exposure to the virus; if R_0 is 3, each newly infected person will pass the disease to three others, on average

SARS-CoV (SARS-CoV-1): severe acute respiratory syndrome coronavirus; the virus that caused the SARS outbreak in 2003 is SARS-CoV; some scientists refer to it by that name, which is officially correct according to the International Committee for the Nomenclature of Viruses, but others prefer SARS-CoV-1, to avoid confusion with the new coronavirus with a similar name but ending with the number 2, and to clarify that these are two different, but related, viruses; *see also* Novel coronavirus

https://www.cdc.gov/coronavirus/2019-ncov/cdcresponse/about-COVID-19.html

SARS-CoV-2: severe acute respiratory syndrome coronavirus 2, the virus that causes COVID-19; it emerged in December 2019 and was provisionally named 2019-nCoV; on February 11, 2020, the International Committee on Taxonomy of Viruses announced the new entity's official name; this virus has caused a severe worldwide pandemic, with many infections, hospitalizations, and deaths, and has created economic hardship worldwide

Screening: brief questioning to help determine if someone has—or has had—COVID-19; often performed before diagnostic testing to make sure testing is appropriate

Self-isolation: limiting face-to-face contact by people who are infected or possibly infected; helps reduce the spread of COVID-19

Self-monitoring: checking oneself for COVID-19 symptoms (*see* Symptoms)

Self-quarantine: avoiding all contact with others by people who are infected or possibly infected; this practice minimizes the chance of spreading COVID-19; the self-quarantine period for COVID-19 typically is two weeks

Shelter-in-place order: a governmental decree to stay in the current location and to leave only if necessary; the goal of the order is to slow local spread of the virus

Social distancing: keeping at least six feet away from others to help minimize spread of COVID-19

Spanish flu (Spanish Flu H1N1 Pandemic): the Spanish flu, also known as the 1918 influenza pandemic, was the most severe outbreak in recent history, with estimates of 550 million cases worldwide and up to 100 million deaths; cause of the pandemic was the H1N1 virus, originating in birds

State of emergency: a threatening situation in which a government can take actions normally not permitted; examples include a natural disaster, armed conflict, epidemic, and pandemic

Superspreader: a person who transmits an infectious disease to an unusually large number of people, perhaps playing a key role in spreading COVID-19; the term superspreader is also used occasionally to describe a major sports event or other gathering that attracts a large number of people

Swab test (viral test): a diagnostic test in which a swab—an absorbent wad on a small stick—is inserted into the back of the nasal cavity; the sample obtained is analyzed for possible genetic material from the virus; a saliva sample may be used instead, in which case the patient may obtain the sample by swabbing a cheek

Swine Flu (Influenza A Swine Flu Pandemic): a flu pandemic that not long ago tore through the U.S. and the rest of the world; the CDC estimates that, in the U.S., between April 12, 2009 and April 10, 2010, H1N1 flu caused 60.8 million illnesses, 273,304 hospitalizations, and 12,469 deaths

Symptomatic: showing symptoms of COVID-19, such as fever, dry cough, shortness of breath, loss of senses of smell or taste, or body aches; the risk of transmitting the virus may be highest just before symptoms develop and a few days after they appear

Symptoms of COVID-19: fever or chills, cough, shortness of breath or difficulty breathing, fatigue, muscle or body aches, headache, new loss of taste or smell, sore throat, congestion or runny nose, nausea or vomiting, diarrhea

Tests for COVID-19: tests fall into two broad categories; diagnostic tests (molecular tests and antigen tests), looking for evidence that the disease *is present*; and antibody tests, looking for evidence that the patient *previously had* COVID-19, as indicated by antibodies in the blood

Four types of tests are available: a viral diagnostic test using a sample obtained by nasal swab to examine for viral genetic material; a viral diagnostic test using saliva to check for viral antigen; a blood test to check for antibody against the virus; and an at-home saliva test

PCR test (polymerase chain reaction test): a laboratory procedure that detects the genetic material of a virus; to perform the test, a health care worker uses a swab to collect saliva or fluid from the nose of throat

A positive result from a nasal swab test or from a saliva test means that the person tested *has* COVID-19 or recently had the disease; the viral RNA is present and the person is infectious (could infect others); a negative result does *not* mean the person *doesn't* have COVID-19 but only that the test did not detect any viral RNA.

Antibody test: A positive test result means the person tested *has had* an infection; a negative result only *suggests* that the individual hasn't been infected with COVID-19

Some infected people do not make antibodies. Others may not make antibodies until several weeks after infection. But, in both cases, a person could have a negative antibody test result, yet could infect others.

Unfortunately, people who have a false-positive antibody test result may think they are immune when they're not. They may stop taking protective steps.

That's a mistake. Regardless of test results—positive or negative—and regardless of the type of test—viral or antibody—people need to protect themselves and others from COVID-19. They need to follow those four key steps: vaccinating, hand washing, mask-wearing, and social distancing.

Antigen test (rapid diagnostic test): a diagnostic test that checks for *existing* infections by looking for specific viruses or bacteria in a sample taken from the nose or throat; although results are available more quickly than with PCR tests, antigen tests carry a higher risk of false positives (they're more likely to indicate *incorrectly* that someone has the disease) and false negatives

On December 15, 2020, FDA issued an emergency use authorization (EUA) for an antigen test for home use that can be obtained without a prescription and gives results within a half hour.

Patient-do-at-home saliva test: the patient places a sample of saliva in a tube supplied in a kit and mails the tube to a laboratory for testing. Test result is available to the person 1 to 3 days after the laboratory receives the sample.

On November 17, 2020, FDA issued an EUA for an RNA test someone can perform entirely at home; the test result is available within an hour. Each test kit costs about $50, and the test is available only by prescription. A distinct and important advantage: results within about half an hour–a major advantage in detecting infections early to help halt the spread of the virus.

https://www.the-scientist.com/news-opinion/saliva-tests-how-they-work-and-what-they-bring-to-COVID-19-67720

Transmission rate: The rate at which infectious cases cause new cases in a given population; *see also* Basic reproductive number, R_0

Vaccine: a preparation that is given by injection, oral preparation, or nasal spray, and triggers the immune system to produce antibodies against a specific virus or bacterium; at this writing three vaccines have been developed and authorized under an EUA for COVID-19, and are being distributed; pharmaceutical companies are working to develop additional vaccines

Vaccine effectiveness: how well an authorized or approved vaccine prevents infection (the disease) in a general population, expressed as a percent decrease in the risk of the disease in those who have been vaccinated

Vaccine effectiveness is determined by 1) calculating the risk of disease among people who have been vaccinated and those who have not, and then 2) comparing the percentage reduction in risk of disease in the vaccinated group.

The greater the percentage reduction of disease in the vaccinated group, the greater the vaccine effectiveness. So an effectiveness of 90% indicates a 90% reduction in the number of cases expected if people in the group had not been vaccinated.

Vaccine efficacy: how well a vaccine prevents infection (the disease in question) during a clinical trial; expressed as a percent decrease in the risk of the disease in the treated (vaccinated) group compared to the untreated (unvaccinated) group

Vaccine efficacy is not the same as vaccine effectiveness. Efficacy is a measure used in a clinical trial to express how well the vaccine reduces infection (disease) in the vaccinated group compared to the unvaccinated group.

An *efficacy* of 50% means that, in a clinical trial, a person who's been vaccinated is half as likely to get the disease as someone who hasn't been vaccinated.

A vaccine's *effectiveness* refers to how well it reduces infections in the vaccinated population. A 90% effectiveness means a 90% drop in number of cases.

Ventilator: a machine that moves air in and out of the lungs for patients who are unable to breathe or are not breathing well; ventilators are important in COVID-19 because the disease can cause severe respiratory infection

Vertical transmission: transmission of an infectious agent from a pregnant mother through the placenta to her unborn child; *also see* Horizontal transmission

Viral load: the amount of virus in an infected person's body; the higher the load, the more likely that person will infect others

Viral RNA: viruses contain either RNA or DNA as their genetic material; the RNA or DNA contains the genetic code for turning an infected cell into a "factory" for making many new copies of the virion; SARS-CoV-2 contains RNA as its genetic material; *see also* Replication

Viral shedding: release of viral particles into the environment by someone with COVID-19; the particles may or may not be infectious

Virion: the infectious form of a virus as it exists outside the host cell; consists of a strand of nucleic acid, either RNA or DNA (but not both), enclosed in a protein coat; some species also have an external envelope

Virus: a tiny infectious entity consisting of genetic material—DNA or RNA—in a protein coat; reproduction of SARS-CoV-2, an RNA virus, occurs only when a virion invades a living cell and the virion's RNA instructs the cell to stop its normal functions and to create more virions instead

WFH: an abbreviation for working from home or work from home; refers to the sudden shift in workplace that became necessary because of COVID-19

World Health Organization (WHO): an agency of the United Nations, formed in 1948 to promote health worldwide; its many functions include naming diseases caused by newly discovered organisms, and helping to prevent, detect, track, and manage acute health emergencies, such as the COVID-19 pandemic, anywhere in the world, but typically in developing nations

References and Sources

Al-Osail AM, Al-Wazzah MJ. The history and epidemiology of Middle East respiratory syndrome coronavirus. *Multidiscip Respir Med.* 2017;12:20. doi:10.1186/s40248-017-0101-8

Anonymous. Coronaviruses. *Nature.* 1968;220:650.

Ashour HM, Elkhatib WF, Rahman M, Elshabrawy HA. Insights into the recent 2019 novel coronavirus (SARS-CoV-2) in light of past human coronavirus outbreaks. *Pathogens.* 2020;9(3):1-15. doi:10.3390/pathogens9030186

Beigel JH, Tomashek KM, Dodd LE, et al. Remdesivir for the treatment of COVID-19 - Final Report. *N Engl J Med.* 2020;383(19):1813-1826. doi:10.1056/NEJMoa2007764

Biggerstaff M, Cauchemez S, Reed C, Gambhir M, Finelli L. Estimates of the reproduction number for seasonal, pandemic, and zoonotic influenza: a systematic review of the literature. *BMC Infect Dis.* 2014;14:480. Published 2014 Sep 4. doi:10.1186/1471-2334-14-480

Black E, Ferdig R, Thompson LA. K-12 Virtual schooling, COVID-19, and student success [published online ahead of print, 2020 Aug 11]. *JAMA Pediatr.* 2020;10.1001.

Bunyavanich S, Do A, Vicencio A. Nasal gene expression of angiotensin-converting enzyme 2 in children and adults. *JAMA.* 2020;May 20. doi:10.1001/jama.2020.8707

Chan NC, Li K, Hirsh J. Peripheral oxygen saturation in older persons wearing nonmedical face masks in community settings. *JAMA.* 2020 Dec 8;324(22):2323-2324. doi: 10.1001/jama.2020.21905

Chang L, Yan Y, Wang L. Coronavirus Disease 2019: Coronaviruses and blood safety. *Transfus Med Rev.* 2020;34(2):75-80. doi:10.1016/j.tmrv.2020.02.003

Enserink M. Coronavirus rips through Dutch mink farms, triggering culls. *Science.* 2020;368:1169.

Estrich CG, Mikkelsen M, Morrissey R, et al. Estimating COVID-19 prevalence and infection control practices among US dentists. *J Am Dent Assoc.* 2020;151(11):815-824. doi:10.1016/j.adaj.2020.09.005

Gottlieb S, Rivers C, McClellan MB, Silvis L, Watson C. National coronavirus response: A road map to reopening. *American Enterprise Institute.* www.aei.org. Accessed April 11, 2020.

Halpin DMG, Faner R, Sibila O, Badia JR, Agusti A. Do chronic respiratory diseases or their treatment affect the risk of SARS-CoV-2 infection? *The Lancet.* Published online April 3, 2020 https://doi.org/10.1016/S2213-2600(20)30167-3

Hermans C, Weill A, Pierce GF. The COVID-19 pandemic: New global challenges for the hemophilia community. *Haemophilia.* 2020;Apr 4. doi: 10.1111/hae.14001. [Epub ahead of print].

Lamouroux A, Attie-Bitach T, Martinovic J, Leruez-Ville M, Ville Y. Evidence for and against vertical transmission for SARS-CoV-2 (COVID-19). *Amer J Obstetrics and Gynecology* (2020). doi: https://doi.org/10.1016/j.ajog.2020.04.039

Lu J, Gu J, Li K, et al. COVID-19 outbreak associated with air conditioning in restaurant, Guangzhou, China, 2020. *Emerg Infect Dis.* 2020
July. https://doi.org/10.3201/eid2607.200764.
https://www.cdc.gov/mmwr/volumes/69/wr/mm6936a5.htm

Halpin DMG, Faner R, Sibila O, Badia JR, Agust A. Do chronic respiratory diseases or their treatment affect the risk of SARS-CoV-2 infection? *Lancet Respir Med* 2020;8:436-438. doi.org/10.1016/S2213-2600(20)30167-3.

https://www.biospace.com/article/compare-1918-spanish-influenza-pandemic-versus-COVID-19

https://www.cdc.gov/handwashing/show-me-the-science-handwashing.html

Morens DM, Taubenberger JK, Fauci AS. The persistent legacy of the 1918 influenza virus. *N Engl J Med*. 2009;361(3):225–229. doi:10.1056/NEJMp0904819.

Ray JG, Schull MJ, Vermeulen MJ, Park AL. Association between ABO and Rh blood groups and SARS-CoV-2 infection or severe COVID-19 illness : A population-based cohort study [published online ahead of print, 2020 Nov 24]. *Ann Intern Med*. 2020;M20-4511. Doi:10.7326/M20-4511

Reynolds KA, Sexton JD, Norman A, McClelland DJ. Comparison of electric hand dryers and paper towels for hand hygiene: a critical review of the literature. *J Appl Microbiol*. 2021;130(1):25-39. doi: 10.1111/jam.14796. Epub 2020 Aug 14.

Rubin R. Sorting out whether vitamin D deficiency raises COVID-19 Risk. *JAMA*. Published online January 6, 2021. doi:10.1001/jama.2020.24127

Salzberger B, Buder F, Lampl B, Ehrenstein B, Hitzenbichler F, Holzmann T, Schmidt B, Hanses F. Epidemiology of SARS-CoV-2. *Infection*. 2020;8:1-7. doi: 10.1007/s15010-020-01531-3

Watanabe T, Bartrand TA, Weir MH, Omura T, Haas CN. Development of a Dose-Response Model for SARS Coronavirus. *Risk Analysis*. 2010;30(7):1129-1138. doi: 10.1111/j.1539-6924.2010.01427.

WHO. Middle East respiratory syndrome coronavirus (MERS-CoV). 2019. www.WHO.int/emergencies/mers-cov/en/ Accessed April 10, 2020.

Yong E. The deceptively simple number sparking coronavirus fears. *The Atlantic*. January 2020. https://www.theatlantic.com/science/archive/2020/01/how-fast-and-far-will-new-coronavirus-spread/605632/

A Request

Did you find this book helpful? Please consider doing something that will take just a minute but helps your fellow readers who are looking for books. Would you please consider saying a few words about what you liked or didn't like about this book? Just one sentence would do it!

Please go to Amazon, and in the search window enter:
clyde goodheart covid-19.

Made in the USA
Monee, IL
03 November 2026

67387236R00108